Rethinking Women's Health

Rethinking Women's Health

A Guide for Wellness

Alison E. Buehler, Ed.D.

Preface with Terry Wahls, M.D.

SARTORIS
LITERARY
GROUP

A traditional publisher
with a non-traditional approach to publishing

SARTORIS LITERARY GROUP, INC.
Metro-Jackson, Mississippi
www.sartorisliterary.com

To Mike, who helps make my dreams come true

"Alison Buehler is a walking (and now in print!) dictionary who has researched how to address women's health concerns at every important passage in a woman's life. Fact-packed, resource-dense, rich with quotes and heartfelt encouragement, reading "Rethinking Women's Health" is like having a Wise Elder Woman to guide you, traveling with you in your own pocket."—**Donna Jackson Nakazawa, award-winning author of "The Last Best Cure"**

"Alison Buehler is a remarkable human being who has helped legions of women build healthful, self-reliant and sustainable lifestyles for the betterment of themselves, their families, society and the planet. In "Rethinking Women's Health," she goes beyond mere prescriptions for healthy living to embrace practical advice and insights into healing, health and wholeness. It is a brilliant gift of knowledge."—**Jim PathFinder Ewing, author of "Redefining Manhood: A Guide for Men and Those Who Love Them"**

"I loved this book and couldn't put it down. Dr. Buehler provides an oasis of wisdom for health and wellness in these challenging times."—**Emily Tarver, M.D. Presbyterian Medical Group Emergency Physicians**

Contents

Section 4
The Wise Elder

Rethinking Women's Health

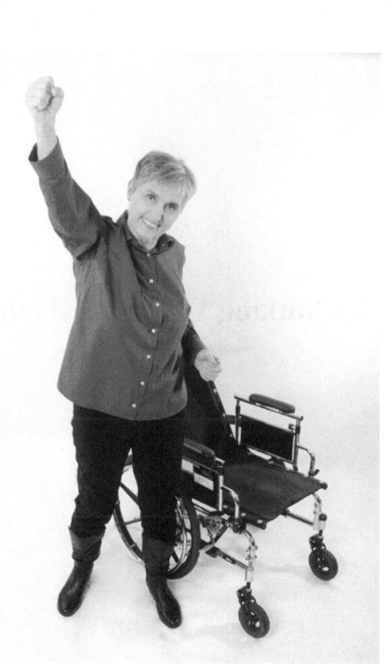

Terry Wahls, M.D.   Photo: terrywahls.com

Preface

Interview with Terry Wahls, M.D.

To say Dr. Terry Wahls is a hero is an understatement. She is a champion for every person who has been thrown a health curveball that high tech medicine and intervention cannot repair. She is a self-described "canary in the coal mine" for a powerful intervention that every American can make a reality—diet and lifestyle.

Dr. Wahls details her inspiring recovery from debilitating multiple sclerosis, which landed her in a zero gravity wheelchair headed toward immobility and dementia. As a physician, she had access to the most recent interventions and was financially able to secure the best treatments, but neither of these assets slowed her steady decline. Dr. Wahls did what so many of us who cannot find answers to troubling health conditions do; she turned to the internet. From her research and self-experimentation she created *The Wahls Protocol,* explained in detail in her 2014 book and summarized in her viral TEDX talk. Uncomplicated, scientifically sound, and widely available, *The Wahls Protocol* is handing health back to the public.

I wrote to Dr. Wahls explaining that my project was a search for answers to female health issues from the very people who found those answers, other women. I almost fell out of my chair when I opened the email that said, "Yes, I would be interested in an interview for the Preface." The following is a synopsis of our interview for *Rethinking Women's Health.*

Why are people so recently interested in "Wellness"? What does "Wellness" mean?

I define wellness as increased vitality and health in the spheres of emotional health, physical health, and spiritual health. People are interested in wellness because the epidemic of poor health has not been stopped by increasing medications or medical interventions.

Did you ever in your wildest dreams believe you would be cured when you began your own health experimentation?

I did not. When I started my intensive diet and lifestyle program I had no expectation of a cure. I had no expectation of improvement. I was only hoping to be able to walk the few feet that I could walk for a few more months. In fact, I had to remarkably improve before I began to hope. I began walking without a cane, but it wasn't until I began biking around the block about nine months into my recovery that I realized I really was getting better. I realized, too, that the dogma that progressive MS only has one way—which is steady decline—is apparently wrong and that no one knew what the future might hold for me. Then, I began to think it was possible I might recover; it became a possibility that with enough time, work at my diet and lifestyle, and vigorous training, I might get close to "normal functioning" for a woman of my age.

I had come to terms with the fact that I was destined to become bedridden and probably demented. Once you accept that, you give up chasing a cure because you know that it is not going to happen. I had to get remarkably better before I began to revisit that possibility. The beauty of my story is that it allows everyone else to revisit that possibility, too.

Why is it so important for women to understand and develop wellness throughout our lives?

Women drive the majority of healthcare decisions for the family. As women understand how to create health and how to restore health, they are not only impacting their own health and wellness, but also the health and wellness of their entire family. If women are putting health-promoting foods on the table and having the family engage in more health-promoting activities, they are changing the health of the entire family unit.

As women, we take care of everyone else to a much greater degree than we take care of ourselves. I was certainly more attentive to the needs of my kids, but I came to realize that the most important thing I could do for my family was to keep walking a little bit longer myself.

How do you convince people that wellness is possible, even likely, if they make some basic changes in diet and lifestyle?

I don't argue with people. In my clinics, I explain that all of our brains begin deteriorating at age eighteen. We begin losing synapses. We can accelerate that rate of loss with stress, inactivity, and poor nutrition, or we can allow the brain to repair itself and dramatically slow down the aging process. Then I ask people, "Do you want to know how to do that, or are you happy with steady decline headed toward dementia?"

If people say they do want to have continued activity into their sixties, eighties, and nineties, I say, "Okay, here is what we need to do." I have these wonderful handouts that I use to teach these concepts, and then when I am done, I ask the patient what he or she learned and what he or she is going to do.

I note the response in the client's chart, and the next time I see the person, I follow up on it. I would say easily 19 out of 20 agree. They say, "I'm going to start; I'm ready to go on a Paleo Diet;" or, "You know what? I'm going to start eating a big green salad every day."

If you have eaten no vegetables and now are talking about eating a salad and vegetables every day, two servings a day, that is almost an infinite change. I'll celebrate that. I celebrate the steps people make. I celebrate that they heard at least part of the message.

You will certainly have much more dramatic results the more you do. If people say it's not helping, the first question we have to assess is how much of the protocol the person is actually doing and then figure out if we can help that person implement the protocol more successfully. Occasionally, we may have to do more of a functional medical work up to see if there are other food sensitivities, other toxins, other infections, or other factors we have to address to personalize the program more specifically.

When I wrote my book it was for a public health audience. There is no protocol that someone can write that will work 100 percent for everyone. You have to make a public health decision centered around the greatest good and the least harm. Then we have to remind people to start here and to work with their doctors, and if things aren't going as well as they hoped, then they are going to have to have further testing and further personalization. However, for the vast majority of Americans, probably 99.9 percent, their health would be dramatically improved if they implemented those *Wahls Protocols*.

You are a physician. What do you think about women looking outside the traditional medical system for answers to health questions?

Oh my goodness, we all need to. The traditional medical answers? We haven't solved anything. We are spending more money, using more drugs, and staging more interventions, yet as a nation, our health statistics are getting steadily worse.

As a nation, we are more obese, we have more diabetes, we have more autoimmune disorders, and we have more mental health problems. In our children, we are seeing more learning disabilities, diabetes, and autism.

We have more cancers, earlier dementia, and less productive work forces. Modern medicine has not solved this. The solution requires diet and lifestyle.

Lifestyle encompasses physical activity, healthy behaviors, social networks, your relationships with your spouse or family, and your purpose in life. Some questions to consider are: What has your infection history been?

What is the condition of your microbiome, the bacteria on your skin, your mouth, and your gut? Are they healthy, or have you damaged them from antibiotic use? Lifestyle also includes meditation. I meditate daily. We start with food, but as people get their diets in shape, we begin bringing in the other aspects of lifestyle.

What progress do you see in traditional medical practitioners accepting and recommending diet and lifestyle as "prescriptions?"

My approach is that rather than tell physicians what I am taking away, I tell the doctor that their patient wants to eat six to nine cups of vegetables every day. Then I ask whether or not we have to make any adjustments with medication, based on this new diet. For most people, the answer is no.

I wouldn't bother telling your doctor you're going to quit eating grains, legumes, and dairy. It doesn't really matter to your doctor if you are ramping up the vegetables and following my protocol. We have already tested and verified that this program is nutrient dense and will help with any nutrient deficiency problem. All doctors need to know is if there is a food/medication interaction or a food/disease interaction. You don't have to tell your physician you're going to quit eating sugar.

I have been talking food and lifestyle with my clinics for nearly seven years, and in that seven years it has become much more common for patients to tell me about someone they know who has changed his or her diet and experienced marked health benefits. People are recognizing in their sphere of friends that diet and lifestyle is making a big difference.

The other thing that has happened is that my colleagues were completely baffled about why I was talking about this, and they complained. My chief of staff called and asked, "What are you doing?" People were getting tense about this, so I had to explain my studies to him. I brought my eighty-five papers over and showed him, and he became very supportive.

Then we started doing our research, and we present our research every year at the Research Week held by the College of Medicine and Internal Medicine. People see our data and the clinical research, and it is very exciting. The clinicians are becoming more impressed with the results we obtain in the patients they send to our clinics. In our VA, we have invited the clinical staff to come to our classes, and more and more physicians are coming.

Our diet and lifestyle workshops have become one of the first recommendations for our pain clinics that are trying to get people off of narcotics. I am writing a protocol to start a study with my rheumatology colleagues because these colleagues have seen positive results with people using *The Wahls Protocol*. The disease activity is way down. We are also launching a rheumatoid arthritis study, and another study for fibromyalgia is being planned. My colleagues are noticing that people in this community are adopting *The Wahls Protocol* and reporting decreased symptoms in a wide variety of diseases.

When will we start to see the power of diet and lifestyle changes become common in our clinic visits?

In the navies, it used to be that you would die of scurvy if you were a sailor. In the 1600s the first navy captains observed that either sauerkraut or lime juice could prevent scurvy, but it would take the official navies of the government 200 years before they would implement mandatory use of sauerkraut or citrus.

In more recent times, we have the example of Barry Marshall who said stomach ulcers are related to h. pylori bacteria. When he first proposed it, people thought the guy was crazy. He couldn't get his papers published. He had a hard time even getting his studies approved, but within thirty years, he received a Nobel Prize in medicine.

Because of the internet, it is so easy for the public to publish and describe their experiences using diet and lifestyle to improve their health. It is easier for the public to read scientific literature and to watch Pub Med themselves. If you are smart and willing to do the work, the lay person can just as easily stay as current as I am on the latest research on the diseases that matter to him or her. That means that the determined lay person who is willing to read the latest science will have the possibility of being ahead of the clinician and just as current as the researchers.

That is very powerful. This new reality will drive change at an extraordinary rate. It will change the way medical care is delivered because the public will go to the health practitioners who use diet and lifestyle to help their patients. If the conventional medical field doesn't respond, it will be replaced by a profession that will help people use diet and lifestyle to restore health.

When I was a young practicing physician I knew that people were spending 6 billion dollars a year on complimentary or alternative medicine. I used to think, "Why on earth are people wasting all their money on this unproven stuff?"

I was very skeptical like most physicians. Now I understand that people are seeking alternatives because we were not delivering health. Thank goodness they had alternative opportunities, and thank goodness we have the internet now so people can learn more readily.

Is there any condition changing diet and lifestyle wouldn't help?

Yes. Being dead. Dropping 150 pounds of sugar (the average yearly intake per person in America in 2000) and replacing that sugar with vegetables will improve your health. Will it cure your condition? I don't know, but dropping sugar and white flour and replacing them with vegetables will give you the best health possible for your condition.

Will it give you the best health possible whatever your circumstance? Yes. If you are also able to add in meditative practice, meaningful purpose to your life, social networks, and movement to the ability that you are able, then you will get the best health that is possible.

For the majority of chronic illnesses that we face, it will probably include a steady reversal of your disease state. If you have a chronic health problem because of a genetic problem, for example cystic fibrosis, dropping the sugar and eating vegetables and sufficient protein will create healthier cells to cope with your condition.

Thank you for your work. Is there anything else you would like to tell our readers?

Over time, I get more excited about diet and lifestyle, and so do my colleagues. The chairman of internal medicine and the Dean of the College of Colleagues are excited about my work. The Director of the VA Health Care System where I see patients is more excited about the Therapeutic Lifestyle Clinic we run.

I understand that with one case of success people say, "So what?" Being a researcher, I agreed that we needed to do the clinical trials. We now have published data. More papers will be coming out, and more studies are underway. We have thousands of followers on Facebook and Twitter reporting success for a wide variety of problems. No longer is it "just one case." No longer is it "just multiple sclerosis." It is dozens of other conditions and disease states. It is thousands of success stories.

Dr. Wahls is there anything you would like to end with?

(Laughs) Hale to the Kale!

Introduction

"The heart is capable of sacrifice. So is the vagina. The heart is able to forgive and repair. It can change its shape to let us in. It can expand to let us out. So can the vagina. It can ache for us and stretch for us, die for us and bleed and bleed us into this difficult, wondrous world. So can the vagina. I was there in the room, I remember."   —Eve Ensler*

At my first doctor's visit after moving to a new town where my husband had taken a job as a hospital physician, I told my OB/GYN, "I have the vagina of Job." For those of you without a Judeo-Christian background, Job is the paramount example of what a person who is suffering looks like in the Bible. If anything can go wrong in Job's life, it does. That described my vagina.

Eight years later, I know my OB/GYN very well and respect him as a physician and as a community member. He delivered our third child and walked me through half a dozen women's health disasters, but I really respect him because he kept a straight face when I announced my vaginal woes in biblical terms.

When your female parts are not right, life is pretty miserable. I am writing this book because I wish it had existed when I was in the throes of battling my own vaginal upsets alone.

Okay, so to be more clinical, the area is more accurately referred to as "vulvovaginal," and reproductive health is incredibly encompassing. This book is about women's health and sexuality in general, not just the lady parts. Divorcing vaginas from sex, sexuality, and human and cultural health is a big part of the problem. Still, my trouble started with my vagina.

This is not the book I thought I would write. In my youth, I pictured a great American novel, but this book is the one that needed to be written. I had been blissfully ignoring my vagina for about four years after finally finding out how to successfully heal that troublesome area, when I stumbled on a Facebook Group called Vulvodynia Support. I had belonged to online Vulvodynia support groups when I struggled with vaginal distress in pre-Facebook days. Vulvodynia is chronic vulvar pain without identifiable cause.

Out of curiosity, I joined the group and began reading the women's stories. They were the stories I had lived for almost twenty years. I began to think about what it took for me to heal, what it would take for the women in the support groups I visited to heal, and what it would take to create a culture of health that promotes women's wellness, rather than a culture that creates and then battles disease. I could not put that thought to rest, and so this book was conceived.

Dealing with female health begins at birth and lasts throughout our entire lives. I started gathering stories of women experiencing many phases of womanhood. I found stories of success, failure, hope, and distress relating to women's health issues from childhood to old age. I paid particular attention to the cultural context surrounding these stories because I believe that you cannot separate women's health from the context in which we live. I also decided to share parts of my own sordid health story in hopes of helping others.

I have been afflicted with almost every female malady known to women. Thankfully, I married a man who has supported me through all of these trials with patience, love, and understanding. God bless him!

Nobody likes to talk about vaginas, hence the landmark play, *The Vagina Monologues*. While playwright Eve Ensler did blow the whole topic wide open for discussion, the play was aptly named. Monologue was about as far as I got with all the dozens of doctors I saw for my issues. I spent years in search of a two-way conversation.

At first I found it so embarrassing to even talk about my vulvar distress with doctors. I minimized my symptoms, hinted at them politely, and always assumed they would know what I was talking about and what to do to solve my ailments. In more recent years, I became increasingly frustrated and angry at the absurdity of my problems' persistence while living in a first world country with good insurance and a great education.

I remember once, prior to children, asking about having my labia removed. I know this sounds outrageous if you have never suffered from vulvodynia or any of the other conditions with which I was diagnosed over a span of two decades. The aging doctor thought so, too. He said, "Honey, why would you want to disfigure yourself? Just take a hair drier to it once in a while."

I was mortified, of course, but more, angry. "Sir, if your penis felt the way my vagina feels every day, you would want to cut it off, too."

I will now apologize to my mother, who has probably never uttered the word "vagina" in the presence of another human being.

I am writing all this on the other side of many of my issues, and probably on the front side of quite a few more. I want to share them with people who are exasperated like I was. There is hope! This hope doesn't come in the form of a silver bullet or a miracle drug directly targeted toward our female anatomy. It comes by recognizing the larger context in which our vaginas exist.

Our overall physical and mental health, culture, politics, religious or spiritual practices, healthcare, and even our understanding of the roles of women all impact the health of our vaginas. In fact, I believe the key to overall female health and wellness begins by becoming our own experts and sharing our expertise with other women.

I did hours and hours of research for this book on the latest "outside-the-box" health solutions for women, but the most effective resources were other women. Women are effectively helping each other become well. There are over a million women in Facebook groups focused on women's health issues alone, sharing their health solutions, encouraging women to keep searching for answers even when specialists cannot help them, and surrounding each other with hope, empathy, and wisdom. For many of us, it may be that stories, rather than science, hold the power to heal. We have so much to offer each other, and rather than handing the reigns over to specialists and drug companies, we need to start taking back ownership of our bodies and our lives.

Finally, I want to do my little part in changing the way culture deals with female sexuality. I don't want finding health to be so hard, so shameful, or so secretive for my daughter or her daughters. I don't want my boys to see vaginas as taboo, or dirty, or worse. I believe that living consciously and making specific choices and decisions as to how we raise our next generation could create a significant positive shift in human sexuality. I believe that if my generation of parents can gain some maturity on the subject and raise our children with the goal of nurturing them to become wise adults, we really could grow a culture of wellness.

* * *

Although this book is primarily directed toward women, I invite males into the conversation as well. Everybody has to deal with vaginas. You either have one, came from one, or are trying to be in a relationship with one. I believe males have an important role in protecting, or at least respecting, female health. I want my two boys to know as much about vaginas, sex, and sexuality as my daughter does. I can't imagine in our current culture that many males would pick up a book about female health, but wouldn't it be great if they did?

You can choose any chapter in this book as a stand-alone discussion on that topic. I have broken down the issues into three archetypes for women, but these categories may not apply to you. You can read the entire book as a story if you just need to know that someone else out there understands and has been through these challenges. You can read it as a resource or just as a way to empathize with what other women are going through.

Many of the suggestions in this book come from an integrative healthcare point of view. Anyone can get the typical medical advice from her OB/GYN, internist, or nurse practitioner. I wanted to cover the harder to find trends and success stories. We are members of the radical middle when it comes to healthcare at our house. We are open to all the options, but skeptical, too. My husband is a physician, but because of our personal journey into natural health, we are much less reliant on someone else with expertise to take care of us.

I like that. I think that the road to health is being able to advocate successfully for the health of our families and ourselves by doing our own research, by looking critically at the latest drug commercials, and by thinking about what we put into our bodies. There are a lot of natural remedies out there that have worked for centuries. There are a lot of bogus remedies out there too. Western medicine offers us freedom from all kinds of heartbreaking disease, but not without trade-offs.

Women's health and culture are vast subjects. This book is not designed as a medical book. I am not a physician. I read over forty books and hundreds of articles, surfed the web for days, and spoke with dozens of women to find the resources I felt most confident in sharing on each topic.

There are suggestions of practices you may want to pursue on your own or with your healthcare provider. I will share some of my favorite resources at the end of this book, but the most valuable resources come from other men and women who are willing to talk about these important issues. I hope this book is the beginning of a conversation, or many conversations. It is designed to be a jumping off point. Teach a class at your church. Start a rites of passage ceremony for the young people in your community. Write your own story. Do your own research. Become an expert on your own health. I also invite you to join the conversation I have started on the Healing Wall blog that shares stories of health and wellness transformations at alisonbuehler.com.

The more I learn, the more convinced I am that vaginal, sexual, and reproductive health are inseparable from general health. The last chapter in this book on sustaining wellness could also be the first. Care for the whole, and you do not have to worry so much about the parts. Create a culture that teaches wellness, rather than treating diseases, and we may really make progress. I looked at it backwards for a long time. I thought if we changed the world *then* individuals could lead healthier lives. This line of thought left me overwhelmed and helpless, but if you turn that belief on its head, it becomes powerful. Our personal choices can impact our health, the health of our families, and the culture of our communities.

—**Alison E. Buehler**

Section 1

Birth of Women's Dis-ease

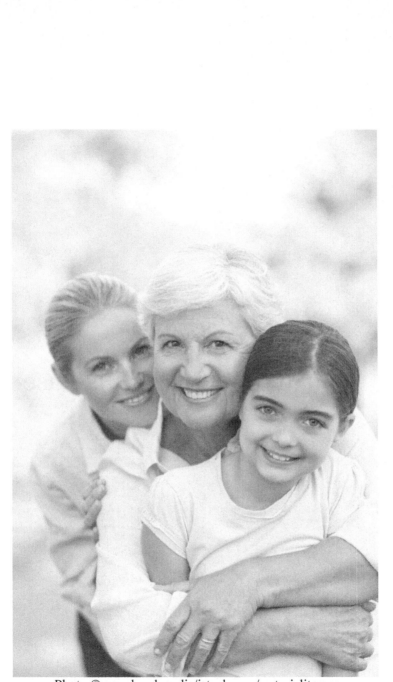
Photo © wavebreakmedia/istock.com/sartorisliterary

SECTION FOREWORD

"So Henry," Puck said as he kicked off his
shoes and propped his smelly feet on the
kitchen table. "I was wondering what you can
tell me about puberty."
Henry turned pale and stammered.
Sabrina wanted to crawl under the table and
die.

—Michael Buckley

To do this topic justice, we have to start at the beginning. Looking at women's health separately from cultural context is counter-productive. Many of our attitudes, our beliefs, and our embarrassment about our private parts set up a culture of disease. Many of these factors hinder our ability to find real wellness solutions. Why is the very thing that brings us into the world such an off-limits topic that it causes problems? Why is it so hard for us to talk to our children about their basic body parts? What is the result of our hesitation to do so?

I believe that we set our young people up to make bad choices that affect their health for the rest of their lives by being too scared to talk to them about very basic issues. By relegating vaginas and sex to a compartmentalized region of medicine and culture, we remove them from the whole context of wellness. I hope that by integrating these topics into regular, everyday life and normal conversations about health, we can heal these rifts.

This section of the book deals with the absence of rites of passage and some of the resulting consequences. I am writing from a white, middle-class, heterosexual, American point of view. I realize that all of my assumptions may not hold across cultures, classes, sexual orientations or genders, but I bet there are some similarities.

A lot of what I have learned about rites of passage comes from reading and hearing about how other cultures handle sexuality issues and how sexuality has been treated historically. Some other cultures' practices seem more helpful than our own method of ignoring the elephant in the room; others are more horrendous.

I find the main difference to be that sex, sexuality, and sexual maturity are at least recognized, rather than ignored, in many other cultures. I believe that acknowledging and recognizing sexual issues may be a good place to start. From there, the task becomes how to reframe these practices so that they are relevant and meaningful in our lives today.

There are an amazing number of online communities that are doing just this. They are recreating initiation rites for young women and men. They are taking the best of history and culture and creating a series of ceremonies that encourage the imperative practice of recognizing sexual maturity in a respectful, integrated, and honest way. It is happening within families and within churches and civic organizations. The number of retreats, webinars, books, and chat rooms dedicated to safely ushering people into sexual maturity and other stages of life is continually growing.

Resources, such as training materials for mentoring young people, are easier to find. This section provides a rationale for why we have to talk to our young people as well as examples that explain how to do it.

Chapter 1
Initiated Adults

"I can't believe it's actually happening. This is independent adulthood, this is what it feels like. Shouldn't there be some sort of ritual? In certain remote African tribes there'd be some incredible four day rites of passage ceremony involving tattooing and potent hallucinogenic drugs extracted from tree-frogs, and village elders smearing my body with monkey blood, but here, rites of passage is all about three new pairs of pants and stuffing your duvet in a bin-liner."
　　　　　　　　　　　　　　　—David Nichols

Elephant in the Room

Think for just a moment about the first time you learned what your vagina was really for. Think back to when it went from being just another hole to being That Hole. How did it happen? Did you hear it from a friend at school? Did your parents sit you down for an awkward conversation?

Some of us were luckier than others. I have a few girlfriends whose parents actually tried to make their transition to "womanhood" beautiful or special.

My friend Lisa's parents took the whole family out to dinner when she got her period. Another friend's mom awkwardly tried to equate her womanhood with flowers blooming and bought her a dozen roses. Most of us get nothing.

I have dozens of girlfriends whose parents never said a word about sex, menstruation, or where babies come from. Never. These girls found out through friends and guiltily asked for maxi pads when they started bleeding. By the time sex ed rolls around in school, most of us are already full of misinformation.

I met a lady recently who said she was supplied maxi pads by a friend her entire way through high school because she was too embarrassed to ask her mother. What in the world did her mom think she was doing all those years? What kind of delusion are we living under that we can't address a very basic physiological function: the most basic physiological function? Why is it so embarrassing, and what are we sacrificing by keeping some warped silence around the basis for life?

Evading conversations about basic human physiology with kids creates a strange kind of vacuum in self-awareness and in health. If our own families can't talk about how life works and how our bodies play a central role in life cycles, how are we supposed to have the knowledge to understand when something is right or wrong with our health? Is it any wonder that young girls show up at the gynecologist with no notion that they are pregnant or afflicted with a sexually transmitted disease?

When my husband was in medical school in Jackson, Mississippi, unknown pregnancy was a routine emergency room phenomenon. A young woman would come in complaining of abdominal pain and—boom—a baby was caught hours later. Granted, there is wide-spread poverty in Jackson, and poverty is often blamed for ignorance or irresponsible sex, but being divorced from our bodies is not an issue unique to people in poverty. We have all heard the story of the middle-class, white girl in New Jersey who gave birth at her prom! I am talking about the issue of an entire culture being divorced from our sexuality.

We don't trust teenagers to get up on their own for school, yet we assume that they can make mental and emotional decisions about sexual health and behavior without discussing it. We expect them to make good choices about sexual health when we as adults cannot even tell them what's what without blushing. As I worked on this book, I had dozens of conversations with friends who wholeheartedly agreed with my argument but still could not bring themselves to address the topic with their own children. Why?

Moving in the Right Direction

American culture is making strides in getting information out to young people. It seems like each generation is savvier than the previous one. Adolescents simply have more exposure to sex, given the popularity of media coverage like MTV's Teen Mom series and HPV vaccinations becoming routine for young people.

Multi-million dollar educational campaigns claim responsibility for lowering rates of teen pregnancy, sexual abuse among children, and sexual assault. Rates of teen pregnancy are at an all-time low in the United States although still higher than in other developed countries. Rates of sexual abuse are declining, and rates of sexual assault have fallen by more than 50 percent in recent years, according to Rape, Abuse & Incest National Network (RAINN).

These statistics are encouraging. They demonstrate an ability to change behavior over time when young people are presented with the right information in educational or family environments. However, despite these gains, rates of STDs are increasing. What is going on?

It appears that adolescents are figuring out how to avoid pregnancy but not STDs. Although the increase in rates of STDs is likely due in part to more sensitive and available screening, the bulk of these diseases is contracted by people aged 15 to 24, according to Centers for Disease Control and Prevention (CDC).

Fifty percent of sexually active people will have contracted an STD by the age of 25. This means that by the time young adults are old enough to make good decisions, many of them will have contracted a disease with serious health risks. Can we ignore those numbers because they surround a subject that is uncomfortable?

Surrounded by Junk Context

Mary Pipher, in *Reviving Ophelia*, describes the context adolescents enter into as a "media flooded world filled with junk values."

Girls understand from a very early age that their most valued asset is appearing sexy to males. This condition is natural and common in most animal species. However, for humans this phenomenon is a problem. Our biology and our evolved brains do not match.

We have decided that as an elevated species, we should have a human-alone respect for life. Nations are founded upon equality, wars are fought about the definition of a human being, and women all over the world battle for their place at the polls, yet our base biology continues to trump the way we treat sex. It remains exploitable as a commodity, monetarily valuable, and one of the most easily commercialized aspects of life.

How do we truly expect to raise adolescents who value their bodies as special enough to care for when pornography sits on the shelves of every airport magazine rack? We tell young women to respect their bodies. We tell young men to respect young women. But when we turn on the TV for thirty minutes, they have to know we are lying.

We are so numb to the selling of sex in commercials and media that we don't even notice. We laugh it off, make a joke to kids: "Uh oh, cover your eyes! They are kissing!"

I delved quickly into, and then back out again, the data on sex trafficking. It is horrifically common in this country. And here is the thing. It isn't "someone else" propping up this hugely lucrative trade. It is people with means, money, and education.

It is my conviction, based on my research, that information alone is not enough. Even startling, accurate information remains powerless if it is detached from our culture, our families, and our dialogues. Sex education, religious teaching, or values education alone cannot combat the tidal wave of junk context in which it is received. It will take the valiant effort of parents, our religious organizations, and communities to take on the tough dialogue of *why*.

Here is what I mean. Assuming sex education or values and

32

religious education don't deter the sexual activity of teens (which it doesn't in over fifty percent of American youth), our next hope would be that adolescents at least make safe choices. However, convincing teenagers that they should use a condom, and then assuming they know where to get and how to properly use one, still does nothing to address the question, "Why do you think you need to have sex with this person in the first place?"

We don't talk to young people about what sexuality is or should be. We explain adolescent sexual activity as a response to hormones, lack of impulse control, inexperienced decision-making skills, or young love. We say they are doing it to fit in or to be loved, but aside from social researchers, we don't really ask them why. We do not ask them because we do not want to know that they are having sex.

I remember it blowing my mind when I met a girl in college whose mom asked about her first boyfriend, "Do you want to have sex with him just because you think he wants to or because you want to?"

I don't think many teenagers give it much thought at all. There is usually not a series of conversations leading up to the time when the body says, "Go!" to contextualize the why of the act.

But what if there had been? What if there had been years of open conversation leading up to the time when sex became an option? How could we shape it for our children? What if sex and sexuality were framed as sacred in a beautiful way, and not as a sin or an STD to be avoided?

I went to college in Mississippi, and probably half of my friends were strict Southern Baptists. I have to give it to the Southern Baptists. At least they talked about sex. They passed out promise rings and held marriage-to-God ceremonies. They held born-again-virgin services and said long prayers to help young people stay strong. I even know two or three couples that really did "wait" until their wedding nights. But I know a lot more who didn't.

Education alone is not enough to help young people make good decisions about sex and sexuality. Moral and spiritual sin and scare tactics are not either. If we want to equip young people to respect their bodies enough to make good decisions in the midst of a culture that contradicts us at every turn, we are going to have to talk about these decisions in the context of specialness, not shame. And we are going to have to talk to our kids a lot!

Changing Tactics

Obviously I am passionate about educating young people on the topic of sex and sexuality. My own children feel the brunt of my experiment and will probably write books of their own one day. My husband is a physician, so we take the physiological approach to sex and sexuality.

In our family, my husband and I named all the kids' body parts equally from the start: "That is your arm, that is your elbow, that is your nose, that is your penis."

We use the anatomically correct terms for body parts in conversation: "Boys, use shampoo on your hair. Make sure you wash your armpits, your feet, and your scrotum."

Except for our daughter, we have stuck with the anatomically correct names for things. Cecelia's vagina became her "Highness" when she learned to talk, and we just couldn't resist.

We also live on a little farm. This helps make talking about sex easy. Every family member knows we are waiting for Herbert the male pig to do his job so Sally can have babies. Our children know what parts are required to make babies.

We have no roosters, ever since Mr. Cock (named by my oldest son) terrorized the kids around the yard, so we have to order new baby chicks from the hatchery rather than hatch our own. You can have eggs without roosters, but you cannot have baby chicks.

Our middle child figured out sex from frogs at the age of five when he determined the frogs weren't riding on each other's backs. We confirmed his question, "Is that how frogs make babies?"

The frog sex didn't bother him, but when at the age of six he realized he came from the same process, he was briefly horrified.

"You!" he shouted accusingly at Mike and me. "You did that? You did that!"

I talk a lot about healthy and unhealthy sexual behavior with my kids. I tell them it is fine to touch their own private parts, but they need to do it in private. I tell them that Daddy and I loved each other enough to make them. When they ask about single moms, I tell them sometimes people have sex with the wrong people, or they decide to raise a baby on their own.

I tell them there are people with sick minds out there who want to try and touch children's private parts. We practice what they should say if that were to ever happen. They ask a lot of questions. I try to answer honestly: "I don't know what made them sick. Maybe someone did the same thing to them, and they never healed." These can be difficult conversations.

There are some great resources out there for talking with your children about sex and sexuality, and the number has grown. Some of my favorite are: *It's Not the Stork!: A Book About Girls, Boys, Babies, Bodies, Families and Friends* by Robbie Harris and *When You Were Inside Mommy* by Joanna Cole.

There are also some really good books on puberty like *The Period Book: Everything You Don't Want to Ask (But Need to Know)* by Karen Gravelle and *Changing Bodies, Changing Lives: Expanded Third Edition: A Book for Teens on Sex and Relationships* by Ruth Bell.

For older teens, Sex, Etc., http://sexetc.org/, is a website based out of Rutgers University. It is a teen-friendly site featuring articles written by teens, for teens, and features accurate information on any and all sexuality topics. Teens can participate in moderated discussion forums with other teens and can access this site from their mobile devices.

For the most part, in our family we just try to make sexuality a natural part of growing up, but our oldest is now ten, and I am about to switch tactics. I have begun to take very seriously the need of rites of passage for young people.

Chapter 2
Archetypes and Rites of Passage

"We live in an adolescent society, Neverland, where never growing up seems more the norm than the exception. Little boys wearing expensive suits and adult bodies should not be allowed to run big corporations. They shouldn't be allowed to run governments, armies, religions, small businesses and charities either and just quietly, they make pretty shabby husbands and fathers too. Mankind has become Pankind and whilst "lost boys" abound, there is also an alarming increase in the number of "lost girls."
—Daniel Prokop

Stunted adults, endless adolescence, eternal children. These are some of the terms we use to describe arrested development in adult society. Evidence of narcissistic living is found all over our current culture. Without formalized rites of passage and expectations that move us along in our development as humans, we tend to do one of two things: Either we will create rites of passage that are more lethal than those of less civilized societies, or we do not develop past an adolescent, narcissistic maturity at all.

Our current Western parenting philosophies coupled with an American ideal of specialness and entitlement enhance the worst aspects of this stunted adulthood.

We enable our children, protect them from any sense of physical or mental harm, and inflate their sense of self to such a level that it leaves them often incapacitated and depressed by its absence as adults. We excuse our children's selfish behaviors and demonstrate to them that taking responsibility for your actions is a pain to be avoided.

I am not suggesting tough love or absence of love is the answer. I do believe intentional love could be part of the equation that encourages growth and maturity. Fostering people into wisdom is important if we want a society led by more than little boys and girls dressed up in suits and heels. It is important if we want a society that is not dragged down by self-centered people.

The Archetypes

In the 1920s, Carl Jung brought archetypes to the forefront of modern thinking about growth and maturity, but they date back to Plato, or maybe even farther. Jung describes archetypes as conscious representations or tendencies. I am defining archetypes as personalities that are generally understood by a culture and recognizable by everyone. For this book, because it is designed for women, I use The Maiden, The Mother, and The Wise Elder. The Maiden represents a period of innocence, but also insecurity, risk, and seeking. The Mother represents caregiving, nurturing, and putting aside her own wants for the greater good, but she is also stubborn, doggedly determined, and prone to exhaustion. The Wise Elder represents wisdom, freedom, and personal power, but she is often marginalized for her perceived uselessness, weakness, or otherness.

The archetypes are not based on chronological age. All of us visit each archetype at various stages of our lives. We move up and down the ladder of maturity and in and out of the characteristics of each one. I have met several teenagers who have lived such traumatic lives and survived that they have deep wisdom to share. I have met women in their sixties who are enjoying the freedom of responsibility like Maidens for a second time in their lives. What it takes to move through the archetypes is some form of "rite of passage."

Initiation rites have been held all over the globe since the beginning of time, marking a passage from selfish infancy to selfless wisdom. Unfortunately, I am convinced that our world is currently made up of a lot of "uninitiated adults." I got this term from Lindsay Wilson, an herbalist at Sweet Gum Springs Apothecary, when she spoke at a women's wellness retreat several years ago.

I rent out our old house to pay for an educational center that we run on weekends when it is not rented. I recently spent the greater part of a week cleaning up after a group of car salesmen and saleswomen who stayed for a five-day training program in my town. I have nothing against car salespeople in general, but this particular group of grown individuals left the house looking worse than any frat party I ever attended. I kept thinking, "These are grown people! Who are their mothers? Who in the world raised them to act this way?"

This instance is an obvious illustration of uninitiated adulthood; people who have not moved, despite their years, into a more selfless archetype. We coddle and overprotect our children in the name of safety. I think, however, because we are no longer asking our children to take risks or do real work, and because we no longer mark life changes with significant rites of passage, most of us are uninitiated adults.

How many women and men do you know who succumb to alcoholism, affairs, addiction, or making and spending money in order to avoid the real responsibility of claiming an adult life? How many adults are able to make tough and selfless decisions and stick with them? How many of us are willing to put up with emotional pain without running to numb it? How many of us are able to forgo immediate gratification? I am afraid that most of us doubt our ability to really get through anything tough, so we muddle by, stuck in eternal adolescence.

Rites of Passage

If we want wise people in our culture, if we want adults who operate out of something other than an adolescent reaction mode, we are going to have to get serious about recreating rites of passage.

39

I thought this was a hokey notion the first few times I heard it, so I will understand if you now roll your eyes and skip ahead. It may be contrived, but I cannot see a more tangible, practical way to help us evolve as humans.

Rites of passage still exist in some forms in our culture, but they are not tied to anything very substantial. They have become rote ceremonies in many cases, or legalized forms of abuse in others such as out of control fraternity initiations. When we do not teach our young people how to hold rites of passage ceremonies, they tend to create more dangerous ones such as binge drinking, dangerous sex, gang and Greek initiations, and bullying. I do not think it would be hard to reconnect meaning and dignity to our existing ceremonies or to create experiences that promote growth. Baptism, confirmation, weddings, funerals, Bar Mitzvahs, menses, wilderness experiences, and graduation are all opportunities to step out into a more mature way of being in the world.

I asked my spiritual writer friend, Jim Pathfinder Ewing, why I couldn't find more information about male initiation rites. He explained that it isn't a Western way of thinking, so nobody bothers to write about it. I told him this was very concerning as a mom of two boys. I want information! He laughed, and three months later he told me he wrote a book, *Redefining Manhood*.

Recreating rites of passage would take three things, I think. First, we need a community that cares about creating initiated adults, a community that values initiated people highly and takes the time to create rites of passage around life changes like the women who are creating menses celebrations for adolescent girls. Second, the initiation must signify something real. For example, graduating from high school often means a drunken trip to the beach with friends. What if it meant young people were now expected to contribute to their family's well-being? What if growing up were tied to concrete responsibilities along with concrete new freedoms? What if children's allowances were tied to real contributions assessed for quality of performance?

Finally, successfully recreating rites of passage would require that wise people receive some sort of recognition and respect from community members. We do this sometimes for a few outstanding youth. Eagle Scouts and kids who graduate with honors receive this, but what about the rest? What about the everyday kid who just needs to grow up and become a less selfish adult? What could we create in our churches, homes, and communities for all kids?

I direct summer camps every year at our retreat center that are designed with an element of "danger." Children come home covered in scratches from the blackberry patches and covered with mud from wading through a swamp teeming with snakes, snapping turtles, and insects. You have never seen happier kids. I keep waiting for complaints from parents, but they don't come. I think we are beginning to recognize as a culture that our overprotection has a price. Planned "danger" or rites of passage hold an important place in a healthy society.

As for my kids, I am trying to create for them a healthy self-concept within a junk culture. The way I am going about this is calculated and specific. I am not claiming to be perfect by any stretch of the imagination. I have as many blunders as the next parent, but if I know what the goal is—a mature, selfless, and maybe one day, wise adult—this guides my actions. It means my kids do a lot more work around the house and the farm than most kids their age. It means we process world issues as honestly as we can. It means we expect that as they get older, they can do more things for themselves.

It means we will have to accompany those expectations with freedom when the time comes and hope we have done a good job—let's see if I still feel this way when they get drivers' licenses. It means that I encourage my kids to participate in cultures that foster their growth, like church and sports, but it also requires that I create some rites of passage that no longer exist. I have a group of women ready and excited to hold a Red Tent ceremony when Cecelia starts her cycles. She will probably think this is dumb, but perhaps, on some level, she will understand that she is cherished.

For my boys, my friend Jim, the writer, is hosting a weekend retreat on rites of passage for men this spring based on his book, and you can bet they are signed up.

How people create rites of passage rituals within their own families is personal. A neighbor told me her son was now a "provider" in her family because he had killed and cleaned his first deer. Her son was not allowed to take a life until he was ready to deal with the gore of cleaning the animal.

Something as simple as girls getting their ears pierced when they are old enough or beginning to wear make-up can become a special rite of passage if you are intentional about it. I often hear "Wings before Wheels" as a saying that means a boy will receive his driver's license after he completes his Eagle Scout badge. It does not have to be complicated, but it requires real effort on the part of the youth and real recognition on the part of the adult community.

Insecurity among families about how to address sexuality with children coupled with what Mary Pipher calls a "junk" culture that promotes a warped cultural sexuality creates devastating health results for young people.

Reinstating rites of passage and encouraging families and communities to foster healthy sexuality for young people is a powerful antidote. I am convinced that if we could reconnect physical growth with actual maturity, we could deal a lot more effectively with the topics in this book. Maybe, at the very least, we wouldn't feel compelled to giggle at the word "vagina."

Section 2

The Maiden

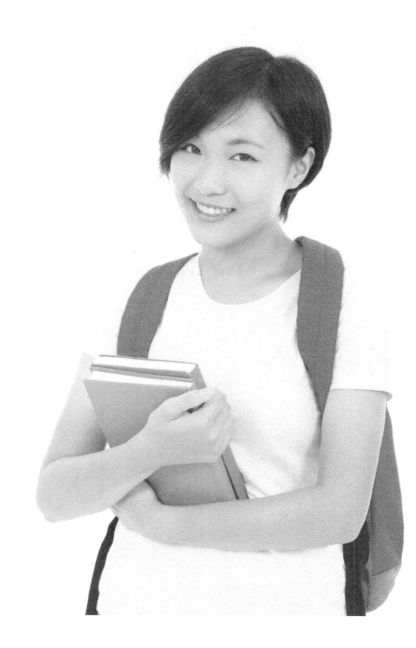

SECTION FOREWORD

"Parents wrongly assume that their daughters live in a world similar to the one they experienced as adolescents. They are dead wrong. Their daughters live in a media-drenched world flooded with junk values. As girls turn from their parents, they turn to this world for guidance about how to be an adult. "

—Mary Pipher

Mary Pipher wrote this in *Reviving Ophelia* the year after I graduated high school. I am now forty years old, and I am sure by the time my children reach adolescence, their world will be very different from the one I experienced. However, I am very confident in saying the world, as it relates to young people and sexuality, is still dominated by Mary Pipher's junk culture.

The Maiden years are free of responsibility, yet confusing. We make a lot of mistakes during the Maiden years, but we also learn a lot about ourselves. My concern is that we are not shepherding our Maidens wisely through these years. I believe that we are throwing our Maidens to the wolves and hoping they survive.

It is my assertion that when we raise children in the context of a monopolizing junk culture, the only way to balance its negative effects are with deliberate measures of counter-culture. This counter-culture includes real, accessible information provided in a caring community of multi-aged people. It means intentional, intergenerational communication and involvement among families and communities addressing the topic of sexuality. It means reframing the value of individual beauty, worth, and expectations by reinstating initiation traditions.

45

This section provides ideas on how we can create counter cultural solutions to menstruation, sex, sexually transmitted diseases (STDs, or as they are now being called, STIs, sexually transmitted infections), and other vaginal dysfunction. I do not believe we can deal with these issues outside of the context in which they arise. Why do we have so many self-help books on great sex? Why do we have so little information on how to bolster our health while we are battling STDs? Why is it so hard to find medical support for a growing number of vaginal and reproductive problems? Why can't we integrate sex with the rest of our lives?

When I was struggling with what one doctor called Vulvodynia, another called Vestibulitis, and another called Vaginitis, I went online to look for information. According to WebMD, there are between 200,000 and 6 million women who suffer from these conditions. Does that seem like a strange discrepancy to you? That is a big range. The reason is that people don't understand it or don't report it, and doctors don't diagnose it. Despite there being a national non-profit for women with Vulvodynia, four Yahoo groups, and hundreds of chat groups where desperate women are pleading for help online from the anonymity of their home computers, no one wants to be the public spokesperson for a painful vagina.

In our junk culture, vaginas are only supposed to be sexy, not painful or dysfunctional or diseased. Hiding this part of the picture causes a lot of unintended fall-out. I hope these chapters will provide a small boost to the counter-culture with which I want to surround my children as they grow and develop.

Chapter 3

Premenstrual Syndrome and Menstruation

"Oh you have a cold? I just laid an egg and now my body is violently ripping down the walls of my uterus, but can I get you a tissue?"
—Anonymous

Premenstrual Syndrome (PMS). Enough said. Until a few years ago, I endured PMS my entire post-menstrual life. At times it was better than others, but for the most part, I got sore upper thighs, cramping, bloating, and irritability five days before my period.

It tended to subside two days into my actual five-day period, which meant I spent ten days out of a month either uncomfortable and moody or bleeding. In the last few years, I started to get migraines a couple of days before my periods.

I had never had a migraine before, and I hate to admit it, but I thought people who complained about them were exaggerating. The first time I had a full-blown migraine, I wished someone would run me over with a car just so I could escape the pain.

I know I am not alone. PMS is a regular part of life for so many women and is so common that our culture feels comfortable joking about it. Doctors generally advise getting on the birth control pill to mitigate symptoms.

Synthetic hormones do work for a lot of women, but many woman cannot tolerate them. Once my vagina was healed, I spent time learning about diet and hormones and how they impact health in hopes of coming to terms with, or perhaps even alleviating, my PMS. I also found some very encouraging practices that helped other women. I want women to know relief is possible.

47

Cultural Context

Getting your period is not a celebration for most young women. We call it "the curse," "being on the rag," or "receiving our monthly bill." Many cultures call bleeding women "unclean." I recently saw an interview with a pilot who still held the superstition that flying with women during their periods was unlucky. It is messy, it smells bad, and it is something most of us just wish we could skip over every month. In fact, many women do skip it with long-term hormonal birth control and hysterectomies.

Within this context, is it any wonder so many of us have problems surrounding menstruation? I am not suggesting a healthy context could cure every menstrual ailment, but I have to wonder what might happen if the entire experience were reframed. What if we created a celebration around young women crossing into their life-giving years?

What if fathers brought flowers and whole families went out to dinner? What if the Red Web Foundation, a member-run organization dedicated to supporting a positive societal view of girls' and women's bodies and menstrual cycles, became the dominant view? What if we expected women to take it easy when their cycle began each month, not out of pity, but out of reverence for the ability to bring life into the world?

In Dr. Christine Northrup's book, *Women's Bodies, Women's Wisdom*, she provides a curriculum for workshops designed specifically to empower girls about to enter menstruation. There are other resources available for parents and educators. Leaders at my church use a series called "Our Whole Lives" with a group of middle school youth and it is excellent. In their program "Faith and Sexuality" sex is presented as sacred, not shameful. Changes in the body are presented in a positive and functional light, and young people in the program feel empowered by their changing bodies, rather than embarrassed by them. What might happen if we altered our view of menstruation from a curse to a gift?

I have to believe that if we change the attitudes we impart to young women about their cycles, we might be able to change some of our physical dysfunction as well. I equate setting up healthy, positive contexts surrounding menstruation to building up our emotional immune systems. It is the old adage, "What we think about, we bring about." If we think periods are painful, shameful, or something to be endured, they will be. If we are brought up to see cycles as a healthy part of womanhood, perhaps our periods could become less of a syndrome and more a rite of passage.

What Causes PMS?

The rise and fall of hormones with our monthly cycles causes Premenstrual Syndrome. There are over fifteen acknowledged symptoms of PMS, and over 85 percent of women experience at least one of them. In an article from *Women's Health Magazine*, Kristina Grish explains our hormones' role in producing PMS symptoms:

> **"The most popular acknowledged symptom is mood instability," Dr. Nisha Jackson says. "Feelings of rage, irritability, depression, hopelessness, and sadness result from a hormonal imbalance." Progesterone (a calming mood hormone) is at its lowest 10 days prior to menstruating. Other body chemicals, including estrogen (which maintains blood-sugar levels), serotonin (a happy mood brain chemical), endorphin (a euphoric mood brain chemical), and GABA (a calming mood brain chemical), also fluctuate.**

The Mayo Clinic's website includes other factors that may cause PMS. While their number one reason is hormonal shifts, they also name depression, chemical changes in the brain, stress, and poor eating habits as potential causes. Commonly, it is believed that PMS increases in severity as women close in on menopause. However, these findings are not well understood. Women's hormone levels don't seem to register differently on tests based on whether or not they suffer from PMS.

An article in the *New York Times* lists other factors that may be involved. The hypothalamic-pituitary-adrenal (HPA) system is involved in regulating stress. This system is impacted by a number of reproductive hormones and neurotransmitters, and disruptions in this system may be responsible for some PMS symptoms. The article also explains that the reproductive hormones play a significant role in PMS.

Drops in levels of progesterone are often associated with PMS. Other possible contributing factors are the stress hormones cortisol and norepinephrine, the neurotransmitter serotonin, and GABA. Certain vitamins and minerals also play a role. Calcium and magnesium help nerve cells to communicate and blood vessels to widen and narrow. Imbalances in these minerals may contribute to PMS, according to the *New York Times Health Guide*.

Why some women suffer from debilitating PMS and others do not is a mystery. It appears there are a variety of factors at play including genes, environment, stress levels, and diet. While the causes vary, there are some very concrete things you can do to alleviate symptoms. There is also evidence that lifestyle changes can alleviate root causes of severe menstrual problems.

Treatments for PMS

While there are several good theories about what causes PMS, there are not many effective mainstream treatment options.

Pain killers for cramps, avoiding caffeine and alcohol, getting more rest, reducing stress, reducing salt intake, eating better, and exercising more are all first-line defenses doctors advise in dealing with PMS. If those don't work, the next line of treatments, according to the Mayo Clinic, are antidepressants, non-steroidal anti-inflammatory drugs, diuretics, oral contraceptives, and Depo-Provera shots to stop ovulation.

None of these solutions worked for me, but they do provide relief for some women. I can't be on the pill because it makes me crazy, but I don't want to be anyway because I had my tubes tied and I have learned about the unexpected long-term side effects I do not want to deal with.

I was on an anti-depressant for years with no results; however, some doctors recommend starting a low dose of Prozac five days before your period, which makes it very light and eases PMS symptoms. I was told about this by a friend and tried it for a few months with great success. I am not sure how long it lasts, however, because I decided to get off pharmaceuticals altogether.

After the birth of each of my children, my PMS symptoms got worse and worse. My periods became increasingly heavier. I ended up having a surgery called an ablation after I spent five days of moodiness traveling in Europe on my dream vacation, and then bled all over a bus in Rome. The ablation is a violent solution to a desperate situation. The surgeons basically put you under in an operating room, insert a balloon into your vagina, and burn off the lining of your uterus. Lovely, I know. In medical terms, it is considered low risk.

The ablation did lighten my periods significantly. However, the ablation did nothing for my PMS. I was told it wouldn't, but I simply did not believe that if the flow decreased, the cramping and the bloating would not also get better, but they did not. I did find relief eventually on my own, and I have talked with many other women who no longer struggle with PMS or debilitating periods. I will share their successes at the end of this chapter.

Menstruation Problems

Premenstrual symptoms can persist throughout a woman's menstrual period and even for a few days beyond. Bloating, cramping, nausea, fatigue, and irritability occur for some women once their period begins, rather than before it occurs. Two of the main complaints of actual menstruation are heavy bleeding and irregularity.

Heavy bleeding is called menorrhagia. It can be caused by polyps or fibroids in the uterus, endometriosis, pelvic inflammatory disease, cancer, or a hormone imbalance. Other causes include a lost pregnancy, usage of drugs such as anticoagulants or anti-inflammatories, or a punctured uterus. A condition called adenomyosis, where the glands from the endometriosis become embedded in the uterus, could also be a cause of heavy bleeding.

The treatments for menorrhagia include hormone therapies such as the birth control pill, injection, ring, or surgery. Surgical options include ablation and endometrial re-sectioning (burning or removing the lining of the uterus), myomectomies (surgical removal of uterine fibroids), or hysterectomy (removal of the uterus).

Women who have irregular periods may bleed infrequently or for a long period of time, or they may skip periods altogether. While we are trained to believe our menses should begin every twenty-eight days and last no longer than five, this is simply not true for many women. A period lasting anywhere from two to seven days and occurring anywhere between twenty-one to thirty-five days is considered normal, according to the Office on Women's Health.

The Cleveland Clinic Foundation summarizes the possible causes of menstrual dysfunction which include: anatomic (endome-triosis, fibroids, etc.); endocrine (adrenals, thyroid, sex hormones, or pituitary gland dysfunction); hematologic (anemia and other blood disorders such as leukemia), systemic disease (anorexia, obesity, re-nal failure, or chronic illness); medications (anticoagulants, herbal or soy products, or steroids); and miscellaneous (depression, smoking, alcohol intake, or sexually transmitted diseases).

It is helpful to start with a list of all the possible causative factors and begin ruling them out. You can systematically work through solutions with your doctor or with a variety of alternative healthcare practitioners. I talked with so many women who, through persistence, found relief after identifying an underlying factor. When a causative factor could not be found, many women found good results with alternative methods or by radically changing their diet and lifestyle.

Possible Solutions

There is hope for dysfunctional PMS and debilitating menstrual periods. The following suggestions come from talking with other women who have gotten PMS in check so that it no longer interferes with their lives. Their suggestions include: looking for and treating underlying causes like fibroids; changing your diet and taking out inflammatory foods like caffeine; starting an exercise program; looking into vitamins and minerals with proven effectiveness (Chaste Tree taken daily causes PMS to disappear in some women); and seeking the least invasive surgical solution. Many women I spoke with thought hysterectomies should be a last resort because the uterus and ovaries regulate all kinds of hormones in the body.

There are also many helpful resources available with advice on how to balance your hormones naturally. These are worth looking into if you have not found relief.

Dr. Erica Schwarz is a physician who has written four books on balancing hormones. She says: "When your hormones are out of balance, you will feel negative effects emotionally and physically. Hormones are used by every cell in your body. You are your balance of hormones." There are diets and supplements for balancing hormones. There are saliva tests you can use to test your hormone levels.

Sugar, caffeine, and other substances impact the whole body. One of my favorite M.D.s, Dr. Kelly Brogan, discusses blood sugar and hormone balance in relation to PMS. She begins with blood sugar:

In the setting of diets high in refined carbs (flour) and sugar, and/or low cortisol from stressed adrenals, control of blood sugar and cellular energy burning may be disturbed. Cortisol is responsible for mobilizing stored sugar to the bloodstream and maintaining fat storage of sugar when it is unused in the blood stream. Thus, when it is low, one experiences everything that comes with hypoglycemia...

Imbalances of blood sugar can feed forward into a hormonal loop because insulin promotes production of male hormones, raises cortisol, which promotes insulin resistance, and interferes with thyroid function and progesterone levels.

Stopping the runaway train requires eliminating added sugars and refined flours (bread, pasta, cookies, pretzels, etc.), and often requires elimination of grains entirely and a focus on "safe starches" or whole food tubers like sweet potatoes and yams best consumed with a fat like coconut oil, olive oil, or ghee. Fats and proteins such as those from pastured animal meats and wild fish are the best antidote to the ups and downs of a high carb diet.

If further support is needed, magnesium and chromium are minerals that improve insulin sensitivity and L-carnitine is an amino acid that shuttles fatty acids to be burned in the cell. It can help with the "hybrid performance" of a system whose glucose metabolism is somewhat derailed.

I have been learning most recently about estrogen dominance. It is believed to underlie PMS and occurs when there is not enough progesterone. Apparently there is so much extra estrogen in the environment, including drinking water, because of all the birth control in public water sources, that progesterone is taking a beating. If the ratio of progesterone to estrogen is off, PMS increases.

According to Dr. Brogan, estrogen dominance is a cumulative load of estrogen that outpaces progesterone, which is thought to underlie symptoms of PMS, perimenopause, and sometimes postpartum psychiatric disorders. The increased estrogen overload comes, in part, from the environment in the form of xenoestrogens found in plastics, pesticides, and cosmetics. Stress is also a factor because it interferes with the body's cortisol production. If the body is in a state of alarm, it chooses stress hormones over conception.

Dr. Brogan recommends several alternative treatments in her practice. She begins with Maca, a mineral and phytonutrient rich vegetable that supports hormone production. It helps the body produce and balance hormones and mitigate the ill-effects of stress hormones. She also recommends Vitex/Chaste Tree herb that has been used historically, and is still used in Germany, to treat PMS. It is well studied for efficacy and affordably. This one saved me! She also lists studies on evening primrose oil and topical bioidentical progesterone as possible solutions for women frustrated with hormonal imbalances surrounding menstruation.

Most doctors will try a therapy you bring to them even if they are not familiar with it, as long as they are confident it cannot harm you. If your doctor is not open to trying something like bioidentical progesterone cream, find one who is. Often these doctors are called "Functional Doctors" or "Integrative Healthcare Practitioners." There is a website called Alliance for Natural Health USA that helps you identify these practitioners in your area. My OB/GYN is always willing to listen to an article I bring in or a treatment I have heard of. He once wrote me a prescription to a compounding pharmacy for an all-natural treatment after researching it himself.

Alternative Therapies

There are dozens of suggestions for treating PMS with alternative therapies. Acupuncture is successful with some women. According to *Women's Health Magazine*, one study found that acupuncture quelled symptoms in 78 percent of women. S. Baker, writing in *Women's Health*, says, "Though Western doctors still don't quite understand how it works, they believe acupuncture may increase circulation and elevate endorphins, which enhance mood and alleviate pain."

I talked with women who have used homeopathic treatments, natural hormone therapy, and balancing their diets to change their lives in relation to menstruation. Herbal remedies and herbal support are recommended by many women who no longer suffer from debilitating menstrual cycles. Susun Weed offers herbal relief for symptoms of PMS in her book *New Menopausal Years the Wise Woman Way*. Here are a few of her suggestions:

1. For women who consistently feel premenstrual rage, use 20-30 drops of motherwort tincture twice a day for a month to help stabilize mood swings.

2. One or more cups of an infusion of the herb oat straw (the grass of the plant that gives us oatmeal) helps the nerves calm down and provides a rich source of minerals known to soothe frazzled emotions.

3. Take a day to yourself around your period. Give yourself permission to slow down and take care of yourself.

The literature on herbal allies is extensive. I have been impressed by the stories of women who have taken charge of their health by learning about naturally available herbal remedies. Most women I spoke with emphasized the importance of ordering herbs from a reputable source, like Mountain Rose Herbs.

There are YouTube videos and websites on how to prepare herbal remedies. One of the most compelling things I have discovered about herbs is how rich they are in vitamins and minerals. Herbal teas designed for women's health are popping up on grocery shelves, which is an option if you are not interested in making your own remedies. Herbal supplements are available online or at health food stores. I suggest doing research on reputable brands.

Diet and Lifestyle

Many women claim that cleaning up their diets and lifestyles have helped their menstrual symptoms significantly. Dr. Mark Hyman is another "outside the box" physician whose writing I find helpful. On his website, drhyman.org, he recommends the following steps for getting rid of PMS. First, clean up your diet. Dr. Hyman recommends cutting out refined flour, sugar, and processed foods. He encourages people to increase omega-3 fats and fiber for balancing hormones.

Second, Dr. Hyman recommends certain supplements for balancing hormones and decreasing symptoms of PMS. I would caution readers to do their research on where to find quality supplements. Google "most reputable supplement companies" and look for reviews. Find a health practitioner you trust and ask him or her for recommended brands. Hyman promotes the following supplements for preventing PMS:

- Magnesuim citrate or glycinate—Take 400 to 600 mg a day.
- Calcium citrate—Take 600 mg a day.
- Vitamin B6   Take 50 to 100 mg a day along with 800 mcg of folate and 1,000 mcg of vitamin B12.
- Evening primrose oil—Take two 500mg capsules twice a day.
- EPA/DHA (omega 3 fats)—Take 1,000 mg once or twice a day.
- Taurine—Take 500 mg a day to help liver detoxification.
- A good daily multivitamin (all the nutrients work together) Herbs and phytonutrients can also be very helpful.

The best studied and most effective herbs include: chaste berry fruit extract to help balance hormones (studies of over 5,000 women found it effective taken twice a day at 100 mg), wild yam for relieving menstrual cramps, and dandelion root for liver detoxification and as a diuretic.

Dr. Hyman highlights Isoflavones from red clover, flax seed, and Chinese herbs such as Xia Yao San, or Rambling Powder, which contains several traditional Chinese herbs used to support female health. He suggests replacing healthy bacteria in the gut with probiotics to help normalize estrogen and hormone metabolism.

Dr. Hyman's other recommendations for lifestyle change to reduce menstrual symptoms include incorporating regular exercise into your routine, managing stress, and trying alternative therapies. He recommends aerobic exercise four to five times a week, but many women get relief from exercise like yoga or weight training. For stress relief, he promotes meditation, and for alternative therapies, Hyman quotes a study on effective homeopathic treatments.

Dr. Hyman's recommendations mirror many of the previous recommendations listed in this chapter for treatment that move "beyond hormone therapy" for menstrual health. If hormone therapy or surgeries are not right for you, I urge you to try a more holistic, functional, or alternative approach.

Conclusions

I drew two conclusions from my inquiry into taming PMS. First, we need to reframe menstruation for young women. We need to stop viewing our periods as something to be endured or survived; instead, we need to start seeing them as an incredible rite of passage for being able to bring life into the world. We need to celebrate and revere menses in order to shift the experience into a positive, normal function of life. How many of us know that changing our frame of mind can alter an experience? We need to help our young people make this change. Second, we need to do the work it takes to support healthy cycles detailed in this chapter.

According to women who have freed themselves from debilitating menstrual cycles, several common practices emerge. Some women find relief by just changing only one of these.

First, some women who beat PMS support overall health through improving and incorporating exercise into their routines. I have a good friend who eats whatever she wants, but if she exercises consistently enough, her menstrual symptoms disappear. I have talked to dozens of women whose symptoms abated when they adopted a paleo diet, cut out refined sugar or processed foods, or implemented other clean eating habits.

Second, some women beat PMS by taking the time to seek out an underlying cause. They went through the possibilities systematically until they discovered what was underlying their painful menses. Take a checklist to the next appointment with your physician and see what he or she suggests in terms of diagnostics.

Third, many women alleviated PMS symptoms with alternative therapies such as acupuncture, herbal support, dietary supplements, Traditional Chinese Medicine (TCM), or homeopathy. This field is daunting for most of us. It smells of snake oil salesmen or "hoo-doo." For my suspicious mind, I find it helpful to research everything I try. I look for reviews, scientific data, or a number of testimonials pointing to the same treatment. The more I learn the more hopeful I become. While I believe a healthy skepticism is a positive trait when dealing with any medicine, I do find alternative treatments with real merit when I look into these options with an open mind. There is a lot of junk out there. We have to become our own health experts and look for patterns of successes, not quick-fix miracle solutions.

Women who have overcome debilitating menstrual cycles say the key is not to give up. Persistence pays off. I found more women who had successfully overcome troublesome periods than any other female ailment I researched for this book. Answers are out there! Our bodies are not generally defective. In balance, they work pretty well. Somewhere, there is a protocol that will work for you.

Chapter 4
Solutions for STDs

"How much wood could a woodchuck chuck if a woodchuck could chuck chlamydia?"
—**Sarah Mynowski**

This chapter deals with alternative solutions for sexually transmitted diseases (STDs). It is by no means definitive. These are pieces of information I have picked up on my search to find out the whole story on STDs, but medicine and science are constantly evolving. The main point is to keep searching.

Your solution may not be found on Web MD or in your local doctor's office, but answers for recovery and prevention are out there. Be fearless in your search to heal and protect yourself. You are worth it!

We enter the age of sexual activity without having much information, other than what is taught in sex ed at school or what our youth leaders preach in church, and surrounded by a junk culture that contradicts any positive messages we might have received. Without rites of passage, or a contextualized positive framework for sexual activity, this experience, more than likely, will not be very positive. Leave it to humans to ignore that fact and keep on going.

Cultural Context

I will save you the gory details of low self-esteem, undiagnosed depression, and extremely risky behavior that make me stay awake at night worrying about my own daughter. I will explain this: I was an extremely unhappy, rebellious young person whose parents, when I was twelve, decided to move my family from a small, Southern town to New Jersey so my father could become a minister after he decided his thirteen-year law practice was not, in fact, his true calling.

I spent my adolescent years surrounded by a youth culture that was trying hard to grow up fast. In retrospect, I have no idea why; all the adults we knew did was work. In fact, there were very few adults around at all. They either commuted to Philadelphia or New York, or they worked somewhere until well after five o'clock. I didn't know a single stay-at-home parent—oh, wait, there was one.

My own parents were exhausted. My dad was busy trying to finish a doctorate degree, and my mom was teaching in a town thirty minutes away. Truthfully, adults were irrelevant at that time in my life. They were like the headless Charlie Brown adult characters: "Wha Wha Wha Wha…"

There were a few exceptions: a teacher here or there, a coach, a youth leader. Since my dad was in seminary, there was some expectation that I attend church. My mom and I chose one near our house, while my younger brother went "student preaching" with my dad farther away. There were some parent and adult volunteers and a youth minister who probably helped me survive those years. I am thankful to them for their time and thankful to my parents for making that community a priority.

But, sex was not addressed at all by my family or community outside of one gym class unit, nor was it confronted by the families of many of my girlfriends. We were young people leading each other blindly through this terrain, which is the reality for many youth in our culture. The resulting sexually transmitted diseases that show up among so many young people are inevitable.

STD Case History

Laura shares a story that is a regular occurrence among many young women:

Before we went off to college, my high school girlfriends and I started going to the gynecologist for the first time. Our mothers didn't say much, just made the appointments. Three of my closest girlfriends survived their visits and described every detail

from the metal stirrups to the medieval instruments lying coldly on a tray. We laughed about the absurdity of the whole thing, so I was not nervous when my turn came. At eighteen, I came back from my appointment with an STD.

Mind you, I went alone to my appointment. It would have been far too embarrassing for either of us if my mother had gone with me. I wasn't entirely sure it was an STD because the doctor was pretty vague herself. All I knew was that I had to go back for treatment before I left for college. I did not want to discuss this visit with my parents. A guy friend, with whom I was not having sex, took me to my appointment. Today, I find it completely absurd that I was more comfortable with one of my male friends taking me for STD treatment than I was with my own family.

I pictured those disgusting pictures of each type of STD that our gym teacher projected onto the wall in sex ed. I was utterly dumbfounded that I had one. When my gym class was subjected to those pictures, I remember thinking, "Warts! That's the worst one!" Naturally, that's the one I got. Later, I understood that they were a symptom of HPV, but I don't recall the doctor explaining this to me. I basically tried to have an out-of-body experience throughout the whole ordeal and pretend it was not happening.

I believe now that my denial was spot-on. I was a fairly smart girl, I understood biology, and I had been raised in a religious context. I attended my church throughout high school. I did not want to be a girl with an STD, and no adult in my world wanted to confront the fact that I, along with my entire high school, was having sex. It was as if everyone thought, "If no one talks about it, it won't be true!"

I don't blame my family at all. I think this is how most young people my age were raised. Our parents were a product of their time as much as I am of mine. I am sure they had no idea how to handle the culture they inherited. The point is this: I had

good parents. I was well educated and middle-class. I was raised in a religious context and went to church every Sunday evening. And I had a sexually transmitted disease.

I was treated for genital warts, and on the surface, I moved on. It was like the disease never happened. The STD came back twice, and I had my cervix frozen in a procedure called cryotherapy that I wouldn't wish on my worst enemy. When the warts came back for the second time, I began a decade-long search for information about something I could hardly even acknowledge.

Prevention

Young people are managing to avoid unwanted pregnancies more often now. The birth control pill and other methods of birth control are now more readily accessible than ever. According to the data, despite the increased number of sexually active young people, it seems that birth control is effective because teen pregnancy rates are declining.

Birth control may prevent pregnancy and decrease the risk of contracting an STI (sexually transmitted infection, which becomes an STD once it produces symptoms), but no birth control method, other than abstinence, can completely prevent an STD.

Again, young people are hearing from public campaign ads about preventing pregnancy, practicing safe sex, and using condoms. Mothers are putting their girls on birth control pills or giving them hormone birth control shots.

Still, it seems that even when we try to make educated decisions about sexual activity, we are still at risk. The United States Centers for Disease Control's Condoms and STDs fact sheet yielded the following statistics: 20-25 percent of college students in the United States have either been infected with a sexually transmitted infection (STI) or have transmitted an STI to their sex partner(s). Two out of three STIs are found in people under the age of 25, and there are about 9 million new cases each year.

The most common STD is the least preventable by the most effective birth control available to protect against STDs, the male latex condom. The human papilloma virus, or HPV, is the most common STD, and no method of contraception can fully prevent transmission. HPV can infect areas not covered by condoms, although male latex condoms can lower the risk of transmission if they are used correctly during every sexual encounter.

Hence, the HPV vaccine is now recommended for all females and males in a series of three shots. Our culture has decided that because we cannot protect ourselves from HPV, we should vaccinate our young people against it. According to the CDC: Two vaccines (Cervarix and Gardasil) protect against cervical cancers in women. One vaccine (Gardasil) also protects against genital warts and cancers of the anus, vagina and vulva. Both vaccines are available for females. Only Gardasil is available for males. HPV vaccines offer the best protection to girls and boys who receive all three vaccine doses and have time to develop an immune response before being sexually active with another person. That is why HPV vaccination is recommended for preteen girls and boys at age eleven or twelve.

There is a lot of controversy around the HPV vaccine, as there is with all vaccines today. Additionally, there is new evidence that counters former understandings of HPV infection, vaccines for HPV, and the relationship between HPV and cervical cancer. The increased immune system response to the HPV infection creates a powerful deterrent to future infection and certain types of cervical cancer. What this does mean, however, is that we don't fully understand how our bodies work to fight off infections and viruses. According to medical doctors Kelly Brogan and Sayer Ji:

It appears there is a correlation between antibodies related to infection and protection from dysplasia (cellular abnormalities) rather than infection progressing definitively to

64

cancer. The commonly held notion that naturally transmitted HPV infection and subsequent elevation of antibody titers is a disease process that leads inevitably to tissue pathology and possibly precancer or cancer, rather than an instance of the immune system effectively meeting the HPV viral challenging and responding with an appropriate antibody response, conferring lasting immunity, is debunked by this new study. Clearly, natural infection not only prevents re-infection but even reduces the risk of HPV's potential induction of dysplastic cellular changes associated with cancer.

I am not promoting or discouraging the HPV vaccine, only demonstrating that there are varying understandings about its efficacy. However, there is significant evidence that most women clear the virus within two years of acquiring it. In the words of Dr. Joseph Mercola: "There are better ways to protect yourself or your young daughters against cancer than getting Gardasil or Cervarix vaccinations, and it's important you let your children know this. In more than 90 percent of HPV infections, HPV infection is cleared within two years on its own, so keeping your immune system strong is far more important than getting vaccinated." He says, HPV infection is spread through sexual contact, and research has demonstrated that using condoms can reduce risk of HPV infection by 70 percent, which is far more effective than the HPV vaccine. Because this infection is sexually transmitted, the risk of infection can be greatly reduced by lifestyle choices, including abstinence. Mercola also mentions risk factors that increase the likelihood for chronic HPV infection, including smoking, co-infection with herpes, Chlamydia or HIV, and long-term birth control use.

In light of the documentation that shows an increase of STDs despite our educational advances, and due to a lack of a clear solution on the part of modern medicine, I believe that decreasing the incidence of STDs can only come by reframing how we teach our young people about sex. Biology overwhelms spiritual or religious training and triumphs over education. Even when we tell kids explicitly about the negative impacts of STDs and teen pregnancy, they still have sex. Biology also trumps technology. Even when we use technology's very best forms of birth control or vaccines, we are still at risk for serious health problems.

In an article titled *In Our Hook-Up Culture, Why Can't We Talk About STDs?* the author discusses the disconnect between how easy it is for the media to portray sex and how ineffectively it deals with STDs:

> **I believe that people are sincerely afraid of the outcome of STDs, because these infections are routinely depicted horribly in the media. But while sexually transmitted infections—all infections, for that matter—will always be something people would prefer to avoid, they're not the end of the world. Most STDs, if not curable, are manageable and don't result in someone not being able to have a healthy sex life or a loving relationship ever again.**
>
> **The trouble with shaming people about STDs and perpetuating the stigma of these infections is that it makes prevention nearly impossible because it makes talking about STDs in a real, honest way nearly impossible. When someone doesn't understand the risk of all their sexual activities, and their knowledge of STDs is limited to what they hear in the media, it's easy to operate under the "It won't happen to me, because I'm not a 'slut,' 'dirty', or 'promiscuous'" mentality.**
>
> **If we don't begin to bridge that gap by advocating for better STD education and a change in the way we talk about STDs and sexual health, and start real, open conversations about STD risk, respon-sibility, and what really happens, the stigma surrounding STDs will perpetuate and we'll lose the opportunity to promote prevention and better sexual health overall.**

Prevention of STDs, or at least lowering the rates of young people who become infected with them, requires teaching young people that their bodies and their persons are valuable, important, special, and worth taking care of. Are they still going to have sex? Absolutely, but maybe they will be more deliberate about whom they have it with. Maybe they will consider more carefully *when* they want to take this step if we surround them with a caring community in dialogue, throughout their development, about the real long-term risks and potential beauty of sex. Maybe we could remove the tantalizing secrecy that makes sex so appealing to young people by putting it out in the middle of the room and talking about it until there is no mystery left but pheromones.

Whole Picture Solutions to STDs

Your doctor can tell you which STD you have and which clinical treatments are available. I would like to offer support and resources you probably won't find from your doctor. I had the incredible fortune of attending graduate school at the University of Arizona in the middle 1990s.

I don't know if it was the influence of Dr. Andrew Weil, the father of Integrative Medicine, or that some other professor got a grant at that time, but our health center was cutting-edge. It offered all the usual services the campus clinic had offered during my undergraduate studies, but it also offered services I had never heard of, like meditation groups, acupuncture, and group or individual therapy methods with strange names. This was my introduction to holistic healthcare. I thought, if I felt like crap and the co-pay was the same, why not try acupuncture?

I probably became open to integrative medicine because I had such a positive experience with doctors at the Holistic Student Health Clinic at the University of Arizona. I began to find alternative solutions to my health problems in addition to western medical treatments.

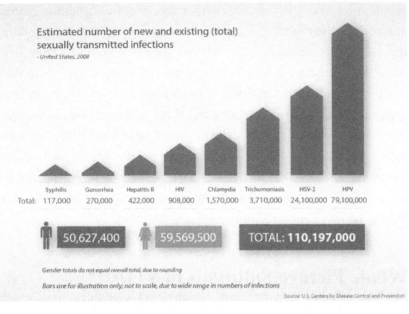

Estimated number of new and existing (total) sexually transmitted infections
- United States, 2008

	Syphilis	Gonorrhea	Hepatitis B	HIV	Chlamydia	Trichomoniasis	HSV-2	HPV
Total:	117,000	270,000	422,000	908,000	1,570,000	3,710,000	24,100,000	79,100,000

50,627,400   59,569,500   TOTAL: 110,197,000

Gender totals do not equal overall total, due to rounding

Bars are for illustration only; not to scale, due to wide range in numbers of infections

Source: U.S. Centers for Disease Control and Prevention

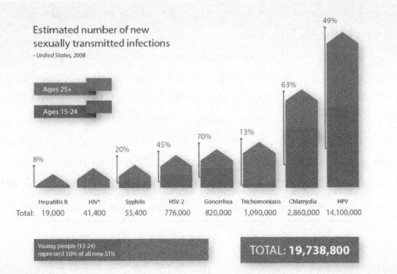

Estimated number of new sexually transmitted infections
- United States, 2008

Ages 25+
Ages 15-24

8%   20%   45%   70%   13%   63%   49%

	Hepatitis B	HIV*	Syphilis	HSV-2	Gonorrhea	Trichomoniasis	Chlamydia	HPV
Total:	19,000	41,400	55,400	776,000	820,000	1,090,000	2,860,000	14,100,000

Young people (15-24) represent 50% of all new STIs   TOTAL: 19,738,800

*HIV incidence not calculated by age in this analysis

Bars are for illustration only; not to scale, due to wide range in numbers of infections

Source: U.S. Centers for Disease Control and Prevention

The basis of all of these therapies is supporting wellness, rather than fighting disease. I am a natural gardener. I know that if I put lots of beneficial amendments into the soil, my plants will be stronger and more able to fight off pests and disease. The body is the same. Although I don't think Western medicine is evil or invalid, I do believe it has made us impatient with the healing process. I believe that we have put our entire faith in the hands of specialists and lost a lot of the "cottage knowledge" that helped previous generations support their bodies at home.

The natural world has a lot to offer in terms of prevention and support of wellness, while Western medicine offers us treatments for disease. Combining these fields of knowledge makes us more likely to achieve health.

In addition to seeing your physician for STD treatment, I am encouraging you to investigate complementary treatments. Getting rid of disease does not equal wellness. Disease leaves its mark all over our bodies, our minds, our psyches, and our images of ourselves in the future. I began to understand that a long time ago, but in more recent years, I have reached the maturity to put it into practice.

Rather than simply trying to rid your body of infection, we could spend our efforts making our bodies hostile to that infection, and healing the whole body from the damage that spreads far beyond your genitals. The body is amazingly resilient with the right support. Learning to love and care for yourself in spite of disease may be an important part of the healing process. According to Laura, one compassionate doctor helped her do just that. Here is the conclusion to her story:

I waited, sweating nervously on the table, for the doctor to tell me the genital warts had returned.

"I don't see any evidence of warts, and your pap smear came back clean," she told me. I teared up in relief, and she asked, "How old were you when you were diagnosed?"

"**Eighteen**," **I told her. I was now twenty-two.**

"**That's hard**," **she said.** "**There is evidence that women are curing themselves of the virus**," **she added. The doctor moved a stool next to me and held my hand while I cried in relief. Sometimes, I think I imagined that whole visit. Until that moment I though this virus would rule the rest of my life.**

It was the first time any of the four or five gynecologists I had seen said anything nice to me. I know that being nice and offering counsel is not their job. I know that the healthcare system is often as frustrating for the doctor as it is for the patient, yet this doctor opened a chasm in me. I wept on that table. It had been nearly impossible, even in my best moments, to feel good about myself knowing I had an ugly virus. That doctor's hand and her words were the beginning of my healing.

Solutions

I am a contrarian by nature. When I talk about alternative medical therapies, I look for the most conservative information. The Mayo Clinic is usually my first stop because, if the Mayo Clinic supports an alternative therapy, there must be a whole lot of evidence to support it.

When I talk about conventional medical insight, I like to go to the other extreme. When I hear hard-core alternative folks suggest a typical medical treatment or procedure, I like to think I have found something worth paying attention to.

I hope this keeps my information balanced. I do not believe Western medicine has all the answers, but I believe it has many. I do not subscribe to every alternative therapy I run across. I like to take the best of both and blend them to achieve wellness. I don't believe we have to subscribe to Western medicine or alternative (or functional) medicine exclusively. They complement each other.

Once in a while, I find that the two branches of medicine agree. For example: Dr. Andrew Weil, the American father of alternative medicine, has this to say about preventing STIs and STDs:

The best treatment is preventive. Practice safe sex strategies to reduce risk of chlamydia infection:

- **Use condoms correctly every time you have sex.**
- **Limit your number of sex partners, and do not go back and forth between partners.**
- **Practice sexual abstinence, or limit sexual contact to one uninfected partner.**
- **If you think you are infected, avoid sex and see a doctor.**

Conservative? It matches perfectly what the Mayo Clinic says. I always figure if those two can agree on something then it must be close to true. I chose the father of alternative therapy and the gurus of Western medicine to demonstrate the similarities between these two often polarized veins of thought. I think we do ourselves a favor if we look at health advice with skeptical eyes and open minds.

Backyard Solutions

The University of Maryland Medical Center recommends certain herbs for complimentary treatment of STDs. However, for information on herbal remedies, I like herbalist Susun Weed. Ms. Weed is a renowned herbalist with over 40 years of experience (what else could she be with that name?) I read all of Susun Weed's work on a recommendation by two friends who started an herbal apothecary business. It is extensive. I received permission from Susun to share some parts of her work that are pertinent here. I want to share her herbal support for what she calls the "Collegiate" STDs:

HPV

If you're diagnosed with HPV, don't panic, and do not agree to invasive tests such as a biopsy or any treatment directed at your cervix. Seventy percent of untreated women clear their HPV infection in the first year, 90 percent within two years.

The CDC does not recommend treatment for the male partners of infected women, as "there is no cure." Eighty percent of men carry HPV in their urethra or on their scrotum.

For both genders, anti-viral herbs can help you drive HPV into remission. And it is important to do so, as HPV can cause cancer not only in the cervix, but also in the throat and in the anus, places that are often not tested for cancer until there are symptoms.

A dropperful of the tincture of Hypericum perforatum (St. John's wort, St. Joan's wort) taken ten times a day for several weeks can eliminate HPV from all tissues. *Caution:* This herb increases the liver's ability to clear drugs from the body, rendering them ineffective. Do not use if you have an organ transplant.

External genital warts, a common symptom of HPV, may be cleared up with the daily use of fresh celandine sap (Celadonium) externally, for two weeks. Tincture is not effective.

Chlamydia

Chlamydia, the second most common STI on college campuses, is a serious bacterial infection that can cause permanent damage to your sexual organs, pelvic pain and infertility. The best treatment is a course of antibiotics.

However, a dropper-full of the tincture of echinacea, pau d'arco, usnea, or yarrow, taken three to six times a day in addition to every single dose of those antibiotics, will improve your chances of getting rid of this deep infection completely, with no relapses, no scarring of your delicate sexual organs, and no impairment in fertility.

Genital Herpes

One in five college students has genital herpes. It is an

annoying viral infection that is resistant to drugs but fortunately, not to herbs.

Ointments of lemon balm (Melissa off.) or hyssop (Hyssopus off.) can be used to counter active sores. Use of both the oil (externally) and the tincture (internally) of Hypericum perforatum (St. John's wort, St. Joan's wort) daily for a month or more can eliminate the virus from the nerves and skin. Make a brew of one ounce each burdock (Arctium lappa) and echinacea (echinacea roots boiled for five minutes in a quart of water and then steeped for four hours, covered).

Drinking this brew daily for three months can remove the herpes virus from the blood.

Black currants have been shown to prevent the herpes virus from attaching to cells. A polysaccharide in self heal (Prunella vulgaris) has been shown to target the herpes virus.

Glycyrrhizic acid from licorice hones in on the herpes virus and causes it to self-destruct.

To prevent outbreaks, try strengthening your immune system with astragalus tincture, nettle infusion, and dandelion wine. Food sources of lysine — halibut, chicken, and goats' milk — are better than pills of L-lysine to relieve the pain and prevent recurrences of herpes.

* * *

I was an herbal skeptic for years. I thought herbs should be categorized with folklore or fairytales. Actually, the science behind why herbs work in treating certain ailments is catching up with folk knowledge. The vitamins, minerals, and other health agents present in our natural world are impressive.

Once I began to understand how herbs worked in creating health, I became more open to using them. I now have an arsenal of herbal remedies in our family medicine cabinet where over-the-counter drugs used to prevail. Instead of running to the drugstore the instant someone in the family has an ailment, I try an herbal remedy first. More importantly, I incorporate herbs into our diet to promote wellness whenever I can.

Complementary and Alternative Therapies

There are some complementary and alternative therapies (CAM) that can help treat STDs alongside conventional medicine. The University of Maryland Medical Center lists homeopathy among its treatment options. They disclose that while there are no scientific studies looking at homeopathy for this purpose, an experienced homeopath could recommend treatments to address underlying health issues and relieve specific symptoms. The same institution lists supplements under possible treatments:

- B-complex vitamins, to boost your immune system, particularly if you have HPV.
- Probiotic supplement (containing *Lactobacillus acidophilus*), 5-10 billion CFUs (colony forming units) a day.
- Propolis, 3 percent ointment, applied to the skin, may help genital lesions caused by herpes simplex virus type 2 to heal faster. Propolis is a resin made by bees. One small study of people with genital herpes compared an ointment made from propolis to Zovirax ointment. People using propolis saw the lesions heal faster than those using topical Zovirax. More studies are needed to say for sure whether propolis works.
- Zinc, applied in a cream to the skin, may reduce the severity and duration of genital herpes lesions.

Acupuncture, Meditation, Stress Management

"For women afflicted with genital herpes, persistent life stress can be a predictor of recurrence," states America's armchair physician, WebMD. "A new study reported in the *Archives of*

Internal Medicine shows that the greater a woman's stress, the more likely it is that she will suffer an outbreak of the herpes lesions."

Given that the relationship between stress and decreased immune systems is widely accepted in the Western medical arena, I thought it would be easy to find support for assistive therapies like acupuncture, meditation, and stress management for STDs. Nope.

The best I could find from anyone inside the conventional medical stage was a conceding that the "placebo effects might be helpful." My husband is a physician. He is extremely wary of "bunk" medicine and over-stated claims.

What he is not in doubt of is the placebo effect. I always understood the placebo effect to be something that is not real, fake, or a trick. What my husband has explained to me, throughout his career in medicine, is that the placebo effect is very real. It is the body's ability to heal itself because it thinks it can be healed.

While the literature review did not appear to overwhelmingly support alternative therapies for STDs, many individual women's stories did. Based on the scores of women I found who reported positive results with alternative therapies, I wouldn't count out tools that could support your body so that it can heal more quickly from STDs. These women encouraged trying meditation, exercise, or even acupuncture if you think one of these methods might give your body the added support it needs to be well. Whether healing results from the placebo effect or hard science isn't the right question. The true test is asking, "How do I feel?"

The most common theme upon being diagnosed with an STD is feeling ashamed, dirty, angry or depressed. However, many women are combining practices to create real solutions. I know of one woman who felt suicidal when her boyfriend, her only sexual partner, gave her the painful disease herpes. She felt like no one would ever want to be with her again and was not finding relief from outbreaks with the medicine her doctor recommended.

Because it hurt to walk during an outbreak, she had a hard time keeping a job for almost four years until she began looking at alternative solutions. She learned that the virus thrives in moist environments and took measures to keep her skin dry. She then began learning about how to support her entire immune system and changed her diet and lifestyle accordingly. Her outbreaks began to come less frequently as she figured out which foods she was intolerant of. She also began supplements and vitamins and has not had an outbreak in two years.

How are your symptoms? How is your emotional wellbeing? What can you do to support your overall health? Every day I read new evidence about the mind-body connection. Start treating disease by believing in and creating a culture of wellness. Wellness includes physical, mental, and emotional strength. Create that culture within your own families. Make health a cornerstone in your lives so disease has very little room to sneak in. Creating a culture of health might be the most effective antidote to STDs.

Chapter 5
Sex

"Boys and girls in America have such a sad time together; sophistication demands that they submit to sex immediately without proper preliminary talk. Not courting talk — real straight talk about souls, for life is holy and every moment is precious."
—Jack Kerouac

There are thousands of problems with sex, and thousands of good things, too. But I will narrow it down to issues related to women's health. For all the energy our culture uses to promote sex as paramount to a happy or satisfying existence, how often does it really happen?

For all the religious talk about women submitting happily to husbands' needs, I have to wonder. For all the effort and angst couples spend on sex, why is it such a source of contention? How often is our sexuality or sexual preference tainted by shame? How often is sex regrettable, unsatisfying, or just okay? How often is it contaminated by former abuse or trauma? How often is it really worth it? And how could we change our parenting to create a healthy sexuality for our children?

Our culture, our movies, and even our religious organizations, within the bounds of marriage, promote the expectation of great sex. I think sex *can* be great. At least it could be more often than not if we made some major shifts in how we treat it. This is a huge task. It will not happen overnight, but it could drastically improve within a generation if we swallow some hard pills and make the effort now.

We live in a culture that portrays sex as "sexy." On videos and commercials, it is always "worth it." I just received a post on Facebook from a friend about why you should have sex with your husband every day. Every day? Really? A second friend thought it was a joke and wrote back, "Ha!"

The first friend responded: "No. Really, you wouldn't believe the difference it makes!" The second friend had nothing more to add to that conversation. She confided to me that she can actually enjoy sex for the first time in years after overcoming vaginal chaos. She loves her husband, still finds him handsome, and loves their life together, but sex every day, she added, is about as realistic for them as moving to Mars.

Great Expectations

Our junk culture sells sex as valuable, powerful, and always enjoyable. Without our conversations and conscious dialogues confronting and revealing the realities of sex, our expectations for sex are extremely inflated. Close your eyes for a minute. Picture a sex scene from a movie. What words come to mind? Passionate, gratifying, desirable?

Now, take a minute and think about what is missing from this scene: Foreplay? Protection? The emotional aftermath? How tired you are from working ten hours? The fight you had earlier in the week? The internal questions about how your belly looks? For those of us with vaginal trouble: Is this going to give me a flare-up?

Are any of those realities present in our media's portrayal of sex? Has any sexual experience in your life measured up to the expectations *Roadhouse* set for a generation of us? Okay, maybe at the beginning of a relationlship, but with time more responsibilities and physical changes lead most of us to re-define expectations.

We live in a media driven context where sex is usually portrayed as mind-blowing. There are a few brave movies that address rape or abuse, but we do not show these to young people. There are lots of comedies that make light of bad sex. This context, where serious sex is always good, bad sex is always humorous, and abusive sex is in an adults-only genre, culminates to form our expectation that sex will be good for us. There is no information present to contradict this reality because we don't talk about sex realistically. Therefore, when it is not great for us, we assume *we* are the problem.

There is a huge industry based on women's belief that they should be able to have more enjoyable sex every time. Popular magazines give advice in almost every issue on how to improve your sex life. My generation of women hosted and attended sex toy parties where we forked over hundreds of dollars to an old lady who drove a BMW and had us sculpt penises out of play dough in an effort to achieve great sex.

If good sex were about effort, I believe most women my age would get an *A*. As younger women, we swapped books and stories and tips, but when it came down to it, not all women found the golden ticket. Some women found it and then lost it once they got married. Some women found it and then married someone else. Some women found it with another woman. For some women, the golden ticket is the vibrator. Others are still looking or have given up. A few lucky souls do get it right, but not all the time, and not with every partner.

Among girlfriends, there is always one who enjoys the heck out of sex. One of my dearest friends in the world is that girl. She is *sexual,* always has been. She is comfortable with her sexuality, and she is famous for saying things like, "Once I have an orgasm, I can have another by just thinking about it!"

Even if every other girl in the room is having less-than-average sex, do you think they are going to admit it after hearing about someone else's mind-induced orgasm? Many women I know simply endure sex as part of marital duty.

The best quote I ever heard on the soccer field from another soccer mom was, "I don't understand women who have affairs. Sleeping with one man is hard enough!"

Satisfying sex for women is more elusive than we want to

admit. I believe we even lie to ourselves in the face of the context we live in where a good sex life is central to happiness. If it is central to happiness, and we do not have it, what does that say about us? What does it say about our marriages? What does it say about our bodies?

Again, I am promoting honest dialogue. I want my daughter to know that what she sees in the movies might happen for her, but more than likely, it won't. Not every time. Not with every person, and especially, not at every point in her life.

I also want her to know that it is more likely to happen if she is with the right person. A "right person" cares about her and her needs as well as the individual's personal needs. A right person cares about her emotionally and physically.

I am not pretending that incredible sex cannot happen with a not-so-good-guy/girl. Of course it can. However, if we look at the entire context of the experience, the emotional aftermath, and the internal angst associated with sex in real life, I think we get a more honest assessment.

Great sex is more likely to happen for women who feel good about themselves. What do we need to emphasize to let our children know the size of their breasts or their penis is minimally important to the quality of their sex life? My incredibly sexual friend is not super-model material, but she is the one of the sexiest people I know. She is proud of her body. If she gains weight, she says, "I'm curvy!"

I am concluding that healthy sexuality leads to a good sex life. If we teach children that sexual gratification is part of life, but not the whole of life, expectations of sex itself should become healthier. If healthy sexuality is the goal, what education does it require? What dialogues do we need to instigate? What conversations do we need to have?

My daughter is five and a half right now. The "and-a-half" is very important. One night we were watching a Ben Stiller movie with her older brothers, and the ladies in one scene were supposed to be doctors. They came out in tiny white dresses and thigh highs. It was slapstick humor, and I wavered.

What is the big deal? I thought. *She is too young to notice. It is just humor, right?* But I saw her watching intently with her five-and-a-half year old eyes, just soaking in that scene.

The women in the scene were powerful because they were half-naked. The men obviously liked the women because they were not clothed. The camera panned in on a naked thigh. My daughter was wearing a dress from church that morning, so I said, "You know Cece, I like your dress a lot better than those ladies' dresses. Theirs are kind of inappropriate. Yours is really pretty."

She looked down at her corduroy, flowered dress and said, "Yeah, mine has long sleeves to keep me warm!"

I don't know if my little interventions will help or not, but I think that night my daughter felt prettier and smarter than the ladies in thigh highs and skimpy doctor dresses. After all, it is pretty cold in the operating room.

What should I have said to my boys who were also watching this movie with us? I talk to them a lot about falling in love and how they should treat women. I am acutely aware that their choices in partners will affect my life for an incredible number of years! They think I am gross now, but I hope I am planting seeds. What information do our boys need to hear from us while they are young in order to become strong but caring men? What conversations do we need to have as families to promote healthy sexual identities and practices?

Problem with Pornography

I have hundreds of problems with pornography, starting with the fact that otherwise very intelligent men and women somehow justify its use. Addiction to pornography exists in the same category of our brains as alcoholism or drug abuse. Marriages fall apart over people's inability to quit. Prisoners are controlled and rewarded by the availability of pornography, usually violent, even snuff porn.

I compare the introduction of porn to the internet to the introduction of crack from cocaine. Once it went online, porn became cheap, available 24/7, and harder to keep away from young people. Not only is it harder to keep away, but it is also often marketed toward young boys in the form of misogynistic content in video games and animated movies.

Where pornography is concerned, the best-case scenario is that young people have an unrealistic expectation of what good sex looks like. Watching the moaning and groaning of air-brushed women for men who spend no time on foreplay sets women up for less-than-satisfying sex lives. It sets men up to be totally incompetent lovers with warped expectations for women's bodies. We would do our boys such a favor if we could tell them, "Guys, good sex for women looks nothing like your videos. Quit being a schmuck and learn some moves!"

If we are not talking about healthy sexual behavior with our young men and women on a constant and open basis, they will find an unhealthy version sooner than we can imagine. A friend of mine has a son a couple of years older than my own boys. He owns his own iPad for video games, and recently my friend picked it up to search for a recipe because she couldn't find hers. She didn't know whether to laugh or cry when she saw a man riding a woman who was pretending to be a goat.

What does it do to kids' views of sexual activity if their first introduction is truly disturbing? Without the preceding conversations about what healthy sex is, how do children have any framework for a goat lady? We have to provide strong foundations around healthy sexuality within the context of loving families and communities if we want to grow a healthy sexual culture.

Think it isn't your kid? A study in the southeastern U.S. posted on internetsafety.org found that 53 percent of boys and 28 percent of girls (ages 12-15) reported use of sexually explicit media. The Internet was the most popular forum for viewing. I urge you to visit sites like *Enough is Enough* to find out how to protect your kids. Turn on the filters on the computers. Talk about how sick people are trying to make money from a part of their brain that is still developing and very sensitive. Tell them what healthy, normal sexual behavior is and is not.

My ten-year-old sat down next to me two weeks ago and looked very uncomfortable. He said, "Mom, you know when you said there are people with a brain sickness out there trying to get kids to look at inappropriate stuff? I accidentally found one. I was looking for soccer videos on YouTube and I found a bad video."

Holy shit. I took a deep breath.

"Well, that is inappropriate for kids isn't it?" I asked, then continued, "I'm sorry there are people putting those pictures on the internet so you have to see them. It kind of makes you feel embarrassed doesn't it?"

"Why do they do that?" he asked me.

"Well, when your hormones kick in, a part of your brain will like to see things like naked people. That is normal. But some people try to make money off that part of your brain and put those pictures out so kids can see them. I guess they don't care about anything but making money."

"It is so gross," he said.

"I am glad you think it is gross still, but one day you won't, and I want you to know that those pictures are just like commercials trying to sell you something you don't need." I said I was glad he told me and that he had not done anything wrong. I don't know if I said the right things, but I'm glad he felt like he could talk to me about it. I feel like our former dialogues opened the way for an honest conversation rather than a dirty secret he had to somehow compartmentalize in a ten-year-old brain.

The statistics on pornography are horrifying, and the content is getting worse. This can be a hard topic to address with husbands who grew up trying to get their hands on girly magazines. Most of our husbands, fathers, sons, and many of our mothers have accepted pornography as an inevitable part of life, and so does the next generation.

In a study examining a population of emerging adults aged 18 to 26 and posted on internetsafety.org, roughly two-thirds (67 percent) of young men and one-half (49 percent) of young women agreed that viewing pornography is acceptable.

It can be hard to be the one in the family to say, "This is not acceptable." For most men my age, internet pornography was a god-send that arrived just as we entered our college years. It was normalized. We will have to be persistent in order to be heard on this issue and to create a counter-culture where it is not acceptable. We can't afford not to.

Remember the rape case in that little Ohio town a couple of years ago by the white, middle-class football players? They looked just like the kids I went to school with. They look just like my boys probably will look at that age. A girl passed out at a party, and several of them had sex with her, then they texted and tweeted about it. Instead of going to college, they went to prison.

"How in the world?" I kept asking myself, as I watched the footage of their trials. So many lives ruined in a single night of beer drinking. These boys were not hardened criminals or evil people, but they had no ability to tell right from wrong. How could they if internet pornography was their only reference? How could they if no honest conversations accompanied what they most likely saw on a consistent basis? My heart ached for that girl in the case, but I felt sorry for those boys, too.

Youth who look at violent X-rated material are six times more likely to report forcing someone to do something sexual online or in person versus youth not exposed to X-rated material. If you *know* that viewing violent pornography, even on accident, increases the likelihood of your children perpetrating a violent act that could ruin their lives and the lives of others, isn't it imperative that we do something? Are we willing to sacrifice our kids to an addictive, destructive, and lucrative enterprise because we are too embarrassed to talk about it? I hope not.

One of my favorite organizations is called *Fight the New Drug*, which is dedicated to collecting stories of how pornography has ruined lives, and how people are breaking the addiction. They recruit celebrities, and the goal is to make porn as uncool as the anti-smoking campaign made cigarettes. We do not have to give another generation of young people over to such a destructive force. I believe we can fight this new drug if we openly deal with it in our communities, churches, and families.

Sexuality

One of my high school friends is a director for Covenant House in Los Angeles, which serves homeless youth. I asked her a while back, what was the most common factor among her kids. Drugs and abusive homes were high on the list, but what I found astonishing was that she said, "Between 20 and 40 percent of my kids are homosexual or transgendered kids."

What does sexuality or sexual orientation have to do with homelessness? Apparently, a lot. She explained that many of these kids were turned out of homes when their parents found out about their sexual orientation. Many others left home because they were too ashamed to let their families know about their sexual orientation and ended up on the streets of Hollywood.

While it is probably safe to say that all children grow up feeling some shame about their sexuality because of our mixed cultural messages, children who begin to understand that their sexuality is not culturally accepted experience shame in crushing waves. This shame plays out in a variety of negative ways as youth age. For example, lesbian, gay, bisexual, and transgendered (LGBT) youth are susceptible to substance abuse and addictive behaviors at higher rates than other youth.

85

In fact, it is estimated that between 20 to 30 percent of gay and transgendered people abuse substances, compared to about 9 percent of the general population, and gay and transgendered people smoke tobacco up to 200 percent more than their heterosexual and non-transgendered peers, according to J. Hunt on americanprogress.org.

LGBT youth also report more incidents of violence at school, including verbal and physical harassment and physical assault. Increased thoughts of suicide are another result of shame around sexual orientation. LGBT youth grades 7-12 are more than twice as likely to attempt suicide as their heterosexual peers, according to the CDC.

How do we raise people with healthy sexualities without addressing LGBT issues? I don't think we can. I fully understand the cultural and religious load this issue holds for some families. We have enough trouble talking about "regular" sex, so how in the world do we broach the subject of homosexuality or transgender issues with kids? I think the answer is lovingly.

As uncomfortable as some families are with homosexuality, if creating a healthy adult out of your child is your goal, it is important for children to hear from parents that they are loved and accepted for who they are, no matter who that turns out to be. The website *Positive Images* has a page for family members of LGBT children. They write: "Despite the fact that a significant portion of the population is gay, American society still prepares us only with heterosexual dreams for our children. The shock and disorientation you may feel is a natural part of a type of grieving process. You have lost something: your dream for your child. You also have lost the illusion that you can read your child's mind."

"Keep reminding yourself that your child hasn't changed," according to posimages.org. "Your child is the same person that he or she was before you learned about his or her sexuality. It is your dream, your expectations, your vision that may have to change if you are to really know and understand your gay loved one."

My third grader came home saying it takes forever to go to the bathroom at school because no one wants to use the "gay" stall. Even though Ben is too young to fully comprehend what the "gay" stall means, you can bet he understands it is not something culturally accepted. We tell our children that some men love men and some women love women, and that if that turns out to be the case for them, we will love them and want them to be happy. Even still, there is the "gay" stall at school weighing on their minds.

With all the cultural influences telling kids that they are abnormal if they are not heterosexual, it will take a lot of compassion from families to help LGBT youth form healthy identities. I love this patheos.com story from a Southern Baptist Minister, Danny Cortez, about what happened when, after fifteen years of consideration, he changed his theological views on homosexuality.

As I was trying to figure out what to tell my church, I was driving in the car with my 15-year-old son Drew when a song came on the radio. I asked Drew who sang it, and he said, "Mackelmore." And then he asked me why I was interested in it. I told him that I liked the song. He was startled, and he asked me if I knew that the song's message was gay affirming. I told him that I did know and that's why I liked the song. I also told him that I no longer believed what I used to believe.

As we got out of the car, I could tell he was puzzled, so I asked him what he was thinking. In the parking lot, he told me in a nervous voice, "Dad, I'm gay." My heart skipped a beat and I turned toward him and we gave one another the biggest and longest hug as we cried. And all I could tell him was that I loved him so much and that I accepted him just as he is.

Raising kids with healthy sexual identities is hard work for parents. It is complicated by our religious and cultural views about what is acceptable and moral behavior. Sexuality makes us uncomfortable as a culture, and homosexuality really freaks us out, but I have to believe for the sake of our kids that it is worth it to go out on a limb and become a little uncomfortable. The common denominator has to be that we love our kids more than our social constructs.

If you are interested in learning more about broaching these subjects with your children or youth groups, I can recommend a few resources. The Gay-Straight-Alliance is a national youth leadership organization with the mission to create safe environments in schools for students to support each other and learn about homophobia and fight discrimination, harassment, and violence in schools. They have an excellent website with resources on how to talk to your children about sexual identity.

For youth groups and a Christian perspective, I love the book *Understanding Sexual Identity: A Resource for Youth Ministry* by Mark Yarhouse. There are also some great children's books like *Molly's Family* by Nancy Garden where the main character, a kindergartener, with support and encouragement from her teacher and parents, feels proud to display the picture she drew of herself and her two moms at Open School Night.

My favorite curriculum for youth is called *Our Whole Lives*, which teaches a healthy, respectful sexuality regardless of sexual orientation.

Physical Realities

There also are problems with sex that are neither in the mind nor related to the cultural context in which we exist. They are physical. There are over thirty possible physical causes of female sexual dysfunction, according to R. Bason and others in the *Journal of Urology*, ranging from high blood pressure to use of certain medications to structural abnormalities.

One of the big issues gaining attention in the last few years is how hysterectomies decrease sex drive in women. There are many physical reasons that may cause women to not enjoy sex that cannot be cured by articles in popular magazines with titles such as "Seven Tips to Spice Up Your Love Life!"

If you suspect a physical problem is behind your decreased sexual response, I have three suggestions. First, understand that you know your body best. There likely is a problem, and you may have to be relentless to find out what it is. Navigating the specialties and sub-specialties of medicine is daunting.

Do not give up if you think there is something larger going on in your body than just low libido. Try a different doctor. Travel to an out-of-town specialist who has good results, if you can afford to. Try a naturopath or a homeopath if you can. Change your diet. Try physical therapy or acupuncture. Find an herbalist. There is no one-size-fits-all solution.

Second, on your journey through the medical system, be careful about the treatment options you accept. Hysterectomies were considered cure-alls not too long ago. Hormone replacement therapies once were doled out like Viagra is for men. Medical interventions do have side effects, so be sure you weigh the pros and cons before jumping on a cure. Birth control pills help some women, but they make others much worse. The same goes for steroid creams.

Third, try alternative therapies. In the years before I finally figured out what was going wrong with my vagina, I did receive some relief from alternative therapies. Acupuncture, while it did not cure me, certainly reduced my stress level. Ph balancing lubricant made sex bearable and decreased the number of yeast infections I got significantly.

Think outside the box about how to pay for treatment that insurance does not cover. I have an herbalist friend who will barter for services if finances are a barrier.

Check off list for sexual health	
Physical Factors	Run labs – get a complete metabolic panel run and look for abnormalities. Have a thorough physical – imaging or other diagnostic tests may be needed to completely understand physical structures that could be interfering with your body's function. Understand how your physiology works: Read *Come as You Are: The Surprising New Science that Will Transform Your Sex Life* by Emily Nagoski
Hormonal Factors	Look at birth control, diet, and lifestyle to mitigate hormonal imbalances. Bioidentical topical hormone treatments and alternative therapies help some women. Research any suggestions before accepting them. Hormone Replacement Therapy and hysterectomies have had a damaging impact on many women.
Emotional Factors	Former abuse, low self-esteem, depression, or anxiety can all impact sexual health. Situational factors such as stress or grief impact sexual health. Counseling, medication, diet, meditation, and alternative therapies such as acupuncture or Traditional Chinese Medicine are all possible courses of healing.

Diet is not exactly alternative medicine, but you will not find a prescription for a healthy diet at the doctor's office. Do your own research on what a healthy diet looks like based on your needs and begin incorporating it into your routine. There may be an answer out there that your doctor does not know about. Be open-minded.

If you are one of the millions of women who wonder why you don't enjoy sex, start searching for answers. They may not come in neat condition diagnoses and treatment packages. You may have to be persistent in your search for answers. Listen to your body. You know where the problem resides. Do not be distracted when people tell you, "It's all in your head," if it isn't. Think through the problem logically. Make a checklist and start ruling things out.

Here are some suggestions for getting started. Begin with your diet. If your overall health is suffering from eating a diet full of sugar and carbs, start there. There are dozens of protocols to lead you through a diet clean-up. My favorite books on the subject are *Grain Brain* by Dr. David Perlmutter, M.D. and *Clean Gut* by Dr. Alejandro Junger, M.D.

Give yourself a month on a clean diet, and see how you feel. Next, once you have ruled out diet, have your gynecologist rule out a physical abnormality. A tilted pelvis, cysts, yeast infections, STDs, and an inflamed cervix can all cause discomfort or even pain during sex. Tell your doctor how you feel. I promise she or he has heard it before!

After you rule out diet and physical abnormalities, ask your doctor for a Complete Metabolic Panel, or series of labs that check your overall levels of things like glucose, potassium, and creatinine. If the results come back normal, keep trying. Tell your doctor you want to have your hormone levels checked. Ask what else your doctor can recommend.

Finally, if you do not get results, see another doctor or try an alternative therapy. I am a huge proponent of traditional Chinese medicine, not because I understand how it works, but because I have seen so many people with positive results.

Answers are out there. It may take time, financial resources, or personal commitment and a lot of persistence, but you can find solutions to physical problems.

Emotional Impact

You have heard it before. The brain is the most important sex organ. It is why pornography works. It is why sex symbols are worth millions. It is the reason relationships cannot be fixed with sex. It is the reason we do not want to have sex after our partners have hurt our feelings. It is the reason that former abuse impacts sex for years into the future. It is the reason why stress and emotional trauma impact our sex drives. It is the reason many women are disappointed by the reality of sex.

Sexual trauma, child abuse, and self-esteem issues are real. They leave marks on our bodies that cannot be seen, so we relegate them to the zone of emotion or psychology. This does not make them any less significant. Our culture views physical issues as real and psychological and emotional issues as something less. This is not true at all, nor is it helpful for healing.

Absent childhood sexual trauma, it is important for women experiencing sexual dysfunction, especially painful intercourse and diminished sexual responsiveness, to examine their relationship with their significant other. Mayoclinic.org lists untreated anxiety or depression as a major contributor to sexual dysfunction in women, as well as long-term stress. What are some of the things that can cause long-term stress in a marriage? Partner disagreements over introducing children into the relationship, disagreements over whether they should live close to family members, suspicions of infidelity, and disagreements over finances, all are possible contributors to female sexual dysfunction.

Dr. John Bancroft, director of the Kinsey Institute at Indiana University, argues that an inhibition of sexual desire is in many situations a "healthy and functional response for women faced with stress, tiredness, or threatening patterns of behavior from their partners," reports the National Institutes of Health. "The danger of portraying sexual difficulties as a dysfunction is that it is likely to encourage doctors to prescribe drugs to change sexual function— when the attention should be paid to other aspects of the woman's life. It's also likely to make women think they have a malfunction when they do not."

92

Before seeking medical treatment for sexual dysfunction, women who are experiencing conflicts in their marriage might want to invest time in pursuing marriage counseling from an experienced psychologist or social worker. Certainly, that should be a consideration if there is a history of childhood sexual abuse with either partner in the marriage. Often, the sexual difficulties are not either/or; they are a combination of emotional and physiological issues.

Sexual abuse is an issue that causes my stomach to clench and makes me want to run someone over with my minivan. It makes me murderous to think of someone hurting a child.

But I know that hatred and anger are not the solutions to this crisis. Compassion, strength, and hope are where the healing lies hidden.

Many people can't do it. Many victims numb and hate and fear their way through life as childhood trauma robs them again and again. I stand in awe of the people I have watched break free from the dark shadow of abuse by feeling all of its awful pain and betrayal, and then growing wings that transcend their pasts.

Dr. Laura Bergman explains in everydayhealth.com that no matter how much time has passed, unresolved sexual traumas can wreak havoc on a person's life, especially in relationships. Relationships require trust and intimacy. Victims of childhood abuse learned from early experiences that their loved ones could not be trusted with safety and security.

Do not discredit your emotions. When we suppress or ignore our psychological traumas, they manifest themselves in physical ways. For example, many victims of childhood sexual abuse suffer from some form of digestion disorder like irritable bowel syndrome.

If your emotions or psychological load is impacting your current sex life, there are solutions. Our hurt psyches will be heard one way or another, so you might as well do the work it takes to heal them.

In myvoiceoftruth.com, Stephanie Gagos writes one of the most powerful stories I have read about healing from sexual abuse:

> **I knew that I would have to go back in order to move forward. I had to examine the childhood that continued to cause me pain and begin to change the beliefs created there. I would have to challenge the monsters living inside my head and defeat them with the truth of who I am. I needed to shine a light on my life and begin to live it consciously and with purpose, somehow recovering from and making peace with my past. It seemed so far away, such a vast distance with who I was and who I wanted to be.**
>
> **On many days it seemed easier to just give up. This image of a woman with strength and character moved further and further away each time I came close to touching her. What I didn't realize is that the journey was not outside of me; who I wanted to be was right here all along. She was inside of me. All the characteristics I admired in others were already the essence of me. And if I gave up and thought it too hard, too far a ways to go, I would end up succumbing to the lies of my childhood and living an unfulfilled life- a certain death to my soul.**

It takes courage to deal with childhood trauma, but there are avenues available that can help transform crippling emotional pain. Skilled counselors have training in therapeutic methods like goal setting, resolving past issues, and communicating. I have heard some of the most amazing stories of healing from childhood trauma by working through these issues with knowledgeable, skilled, and compassionate therapists.

Adults who have been trapped by a childhood nightmare for decades are finally able to heal and claim joyful lives. The method I hear most about recently from friends of mine who counsel is called

EMDR (Eye Movement Desensitization and Reprocessing Therapy). There are dozens of other methods, and it is important to find the one you are most comfortable with.

However, if counseling is not for you or it is not in your budget, forming a women's support circle or visiting support groups or clergymen and women are valid alternatives. Regular prayer and meditation are also methods that help people move out of trauma to a place of healing. My favorite guide to emotional healing is from James S. Gordon's book *Unstuck*. I also recommend *The Sexual Healing Journey: A Guide for Survivors of Sexual Abuse* by Wendy Maltz. If you are in a relationship with someone who was sexually abused, I recommend *Allies in Healing: When the Person You Love Was Sexually Abused* by Laura Davis.

The best book I can recommend for healing childhood trauma is Donna Jackson Nakazawa's latest release, *Childhood Disrupted: How your Biography Becomes Your Biography, and How You Can Heal*. It covers dozens of tools for healing.

There is no easy path. Dealing with emotional and psychological hurt is painful, but avoiding it simply drags out that pain and gives it power over your life that it does not deserve. Do the work. Heal the hurt. As my friend Lindsay says, "The only way out is through." I cheer like a crazy women for those people who transform their lives from victims into heroes.

Putting Sex in Context

There is a history of "women's hysteria" that I want to touch on here. What I find frustrating is the trend in Western medicine to blame women's sexual dysfunction on our psychology. While writing this section of the book, I did hundreds of online searches for the most up-to-date information for successfully helping women who encounter sexual problems. The majority of sites suggested anti-depressants and counseling among their top solutions.

I am not arguing that these methods are not valid or even

unimportant, but I am discouraged by how they place the "problem" in the mind of the individual female, rather than placing it in the body or recognizing it as a symptom of our larger junk culture context.

I believe that less-than-satisfying sexual experiences come from very real sources. Inflated and unrealistic expectations, childhood trauma, physical disorders, and an insatiable pornography industry create an emotional impact with significant consequences. Emotional and physical reasons exist for sexual dysfunction, and simply relegating them to the "mind" is not a helpful solution in a society that hands out antidepressants like candy.

At the risk of sounding dismissive, if our partners are learning sexual technique from pornography, we will probably need medication and counseling. If our junk culture teaches men and women that sex is always sexy, we will be left emotionally empty from the experience. If our medical options send us straight to the psychiatrist, without taking the time to understand the body as a whole, it seems likely that we will suffer from unsatisfactory results when it comes to our sexual lives.

Emotional traumas are real. They impact our sex lives in significant ways, but not every occurrence of sexual trouble exists in our brains or our psyches. It is up to us to know ourselves well enough to tell the difference. It is up to us to create a context for our children where the junk is exposed for what it is and replaced with a culture that supports whole people who value healthy sexuality.

Chapter 6

Yeasts and Other Vaginal Beasts

"There are a huge number of yeast infections in this county. Probably because we're downriver from that old bread factory"
—Dwight Schrute

Culturally and medically, we have relegated vaginal problems to the vagina. We treat the body as separate parts, rather than parts of a whole, and the vagina is one part we do not like to deal with. When medicine cannot provide answers, it tends to move vaginal problems to the head. Woman after woman has said, "When the doctors couldn't help me, they told me it was all in my head."

It is not in your head, and it is. It is in your vagina, or your uterus, or your ovaries, or your vulva, and it isn't. The problem, I believe, after speaking with hundreds of women who have healed from female health disorders, is in our whole bodies—mind, body, and spirit. This is my chapter. I am the owner of a healed vagina. I looked to experts for years without respite or relief.

I am an expert on dysfunctional vaginas, but I am also an expert on a fully functioning, healthy one. I hope I can share some hope with you if you are among the vaginally afflicted. My recommendations, from spending months speaking with women who have healed, are at the end of this chapter.

The key to women's health is becoming our own experts. Women are not finding many long-term solutions to chronic female disorders in doctors' offices; although, it is important to keep an eye on the latest medical developments.

We are finding solutions in conversations with each other: one tip, one suggestion for relief, one book recommendation, and one success story at a time.

97

For readers who are not afflicted with these types of disorders, please read the posts below from the vulvodynia, interstitial cystitis, and vestibulitis support groups so that you understand why this issue is so important:

"Has anybody ever been in so much pain they couldn't think straight and had to remind themselves to breathe?"—**Anonymous**

"One of the fun things that goes along with vestibulitis: being so used to dealing with urinary pain that it takes blood in your urine for you to think that day's worth of pain may actually be an infection. Sitting in Urgent Care at the moment..."—**Anonymous**

"My specialist told me I might need a vestibulectomy. That area on me is very thin, red, and raw. It has been causing chronic pain for about a year. She diagnosed me with vulvodynia. I already have IC, chronic UTI's [sic] and vaginal infections. Can someone please explain to me about the vestibulectomy surgery?"—**Anonymous**

"Hello, ladies! Thank you for allowing me to join the group. I just want to share what brought me here. I'm not even sure how long I've had these symptoms. Since I got on birth control at 16 (I'm 27 now), I've had frequent yeast infections. I've had burning/itching with no apparent medical reason. My symptoms have gotten so bad recently that I am FED UP with my doctors (primary, gynecologist, dermatologist) telling me there's nothing wrong. Just because all the tests came back negative does not mean I'm not experiencing these symptoms, which are: severe burning (almost feels like it is tearing) at the bottom of the opening during initial penetration, and then a dull burning on the outside only during intercourse. And then after sex, it feels swollen and like there is a lot of pressure. It will then burn and feel raw for at least a day after. It will be sensitive when I wipe or sit a certain way. I've been tested a ridiculous amount of times for yeast and other infections, but have been negative for a long time. We aren't using condoms, so it's not an allergy to that. I THINK there's enough lubrication. I use all hypoallergenic soaps/detergents. So, after hours of research, I found Vestibulitis and am convinced that is what is happening. I am looking forward to learning more about this from you all. Initially, I'd like to know some tips for how to get my gynecologist to take this seriously. And any tips for how to make sex more comfortable. I HATE having sex. Thanks for reading and in advance for your help and guidance!"—**Anonymous**

"Once you seal and heal the gut, which is what mega dosing on fermented foods helps to accomplish, the autoimmune disorders start to disappear. There is a spectrum of how serious it is, of course. Even after 15 years of wanting to claw my vagina out, it only took three months to get some relief from the cultured foods and six months to become "normal."

"I still incorporate them into my diet regularly because I NEVER want that horror to come back. But it wasn't until I really worked on sealing and healing the gut, due to something totally unrelated (my daughter had severe food allergies), that all my autoimmune stuff started to disappear. I never even connected it all before then. I think it is part of the problem.

"Western medicine looks at people in parts, when really the whole body is interconnected. Anyway, I haven't visited this landscape for so long now that it absolutely breaks my heart to read how much physical and emotional pain everyone is in. I just pray for hope and peace for everyone on these pages."—**Alison Buehler**

A History of Yeast

Mary's story is common—unrelenting yeast infections for years beginning in her teens. She says:

> **I am not sure when my vagina started bothering me. I think I was around 14 or 15 years old. It was pre-sexual activity. As a young child I had had lots of bladder infections. I never said anything about my uncomfortable vagina to my parents. It would have been too embarrassing. So I guess from about fourteen on, my vagina was irritated most of the time. The earliest pain was probably a yeast infection. I don't know if my body cured it and I got others or if I had just one long, undiagnosed yeast infection.**

There were periods of relief in between irritation. I did start buying Monistat on my own by recommendation from my friends. This was pre-internet, so I couldn't just get online and look up my symptoms.

My freshman year in college, I went to a gynecologist and the doctor told me I had a "raging yeast infection." I took my Diflucan and my Monistat home with me and got some relief for a little while. The next month I felt irritated again. I went to the doctor six months later, and had another yeast infection. This whole year is pretty fuzzy in my mind. I have to think very hard to recall the details. It was my first year at college, away from everyone I knew and I was miserable.

Sophomore year, the gynecologist put me on two doses of Diflucan a month to prevent and treat my inevitable yeast infections. It seemed to work for a while. By the time I was twenty, I had been to four gynecologists and a few student health nurses, and no one could help me.

* * *

Mary's story mirrors my own very closely. I stayed miserable with yeast infections throughout college. It astounds me how extremely divorced I was from my body during this time. I made very few connections between my lifestyle and my vaginal woes. After all, I lived with lots of other young women whose lifestyles were identical to mine, and they had no issues with their vaginas other than the infrequent yeast or urinary tract infection. Everybody I knew was eating junk food, drinking too much, and having sex (well, except for a very few of my more dedicated Baptist friends). Welcome to College USA during the 1990s.

It was not until I moved out to Arizona for Graduate School and had the fortune of making an appointment at the Holistic Student Health Clinic that I began to entertain solutions other than medication for vaginal distress. I did entertain an antidepressant, a silver bullet called Effexor, that probably saved me mentally, but was not without long-term consequences. I am lucky. Almost twenty years later I know so much more about what our bodies and minds need to thrive. In my early twenties, I knew next to nothing. I cannot explain how I came through that time with two degrees and a body left intact. I am a person of faith, and I can only guess that God carried me. But that is another story.

With my mind and spirit functioning again for the first time in years, I moved back to Mississippi and immediately met my husband. These were the best years of my life outside of childhood. It was probably the first time I had enough good chemicals reaching my brain at the same time.

I was surrounded by friends from college, living near my brother, in a good relationship with my parents, making a difference with kids in a very tough school, and in love with the man I wanted to spend the rest of my life with.

The yeast infections returned, but my mental status was so good that I could deal with them and move on. And so we dated, fell in love, and had a beautiful wedding surrounded by friends and family. The day after our wedding I moved with Mike to Knoxville, Tennessee, where he was doing a residency in radiology, and I began my doctoral program in educational administration. Just like the fairy tale, except the fairy tale stops with the drive into the sunset. Real life just begins again once the carriage parks.

Treatments for Yeast Infections

While it frustrated me to no end when doctors would ask, "Have you switched your detergent?" or "Are you wiping from front to back?" I feel like I have to include these recommendations. I tried every non-allergenic detergent, toilet paper, tampon, and underwear available to mankind. I used non-allergenic soap, and there was no cleaner vagina than mine. I never douched or wore a bathing suit for more than five minutes after swimming. None of these suggestions made a bit of difference. If you are one of the lucky women who have found success with these options, I would love to hear from you. There may be brands out there today that do make a difference.

According to the Mayo Clinic, there are short-term and long-term treatments. Short-term treatments include: a one-time one-to-three-day regimen of antifungal cream, tablet, or suppository, which clears a yeast infection in most cases. There are also single-dose antifungal oral medications (fluconazole or Diflucan). Make a follow-up appointment if all your symptoms are not gone or if they return within two months. Long-course treatments for complicated or persistent yeast infections include an azole medication in the form of cream, tablet, or suppository for 7-14 days. Multi-dose treatment of oral medication may also be prescribed. This treatment is not recommended for pregnant women.

A maintenance plan to keep yeast in check might be recommended. This plan usually includes fluconazole tablets taken by mouth once or twice a week for six months. Some doctors prescribe clotrimazole as a vaginal tablet used once a week. Some doctors also treat your sexual partner for yeast.

Alternative treatments from the Mayo Clinic include using a boric acid suppository (available by prescriptions), which may help if you do not respond to regular treatment. Boric acid may be effective against the less common strains of candida and candida that's become resistant to azole medications. However, boric acid can irritate your skin. Yogurt is also recommended, and is to be taken by mouth or applied vaginally. Studies that showed yogurt to be effective for reducing vaginal yeast cultures and providing symptom relief were done in a small number of women, with no control groups.

If you are reading this chapter, most likely you have tried all the interventions albeit unsuccessfully. I want to offer some advice in the section below for those of us who do not respond to traditional treatment for yeast.

Alternative Suggestions

If you only have a yeast infection or two a year, using Diflucan or an over-the-counter anti-fungal is probably fine, but if you get four or more in a year, something else is probably unbalanced. There is a reason yeast infections are more common among people with diabetes

Yeast loves sugar. Ultimately, diet is the best cure I can recommend, but it is also the hardest. Lots of women I know have had success with hormonal birth control implants because their yeast infections were tied to the rise and fall of hormone levels related to their periods. The implant stops periods altogether and provides a steady supply of hormones. I believe the overall negative health impacts make this option troublesome, which we will discuss later, but if you are among the desperate, it might be a choice.

Make sure you absolutely need antibiotics before you take them. Antibiotics wipe out all the good probiotics along with the bad ones. Once the probiotics are gone, the yeast takes over. I recommend AZO homeopathic yeast medicine. You can get it at any pharmacy. I do not know how it works, but it eases the symptoms dramatically.

Clean up your diet. Cutting way down on sugar starves the yeast. Carbs are full of sugar that yeast loves. Get rid of them. Megadose yourself with probiotic foods (sugar-loaded, store-bought yogurt does not count). Supplements are okay once you get rebalanced, but fermented food that is full of probiotics seems to be much more effective more quickly.

The minute you feel a yeast infection coming on, apply plain kefir or plain yogurt to the entire vulva and inside the vaginal canal or use vaginal probiotics. I know it sounds awful, but I'll give a longer explanation in the next section. Also, garlic is a strong anti-microbial. It kills all kinds of unwanted growth, but it really hates yeast. Incorporate it into your diet regularly.

Finally, get rid of sugar. Sugar feeds yeast, and we eat way too much of it. The statistics on how much sugar Americans today eat compared with two generations ago are staggering, and we are seeing the effects in our bodies.

Learn how to make just one fermented food you love and eat a little every day. Kefir, sauerkraut, even pickles (if you make them yourself without all the sugar), and kombucha are a few of my favorites. I don't have a lot of time to make these, but my neighbor is a fermenting nut. I care for her animals when she goes on vacation in return for weekly supplies of her latest fermented experiment.

Vaginitis, Vestibulitis and Vulvodynia

The first few years of marriage, for me, were magical in some ways, and a harsh run-in with reality in others. The fairy tale had been misleading. It wasn't happily ever after, but it was an adventure moving off and being connected to one other person for support. Mike and I were a team against graduate school, in making new friends, and in caring for each other in a new place.

The first year of our marriage, my health took a bad turn. I began testing negative for yeast, yet I still felt like I had a yeast infection. I felt like a failure as a spouse. Thankfully, Mike is about the most patient human I have ever met. I don't know how he put up with what must have been an extremely disappointing start to our marriage, but he did.

In my mind I wanted to be intimate with my husband, but the physical symptoms sex caused were unbearable. Older, more confident, and more fed up, I decided to figure out what the problem was with my vagina and get it fixed. My first attempt was at the University of Tennessee Medical Center, where Mike was a resident.

Mike asked around to find out which gynecologist was the very best. Dr. Gupta had the strongest reputation for solving tough cases and thinking outside the box. I asked for an extended appointment, which the receptionist did not understand over the phone. "I need to tell the doctor my background," I pleaded.

"Yes, we have forms you can fill out in the waiting room."

"Yes Ma'am, I know about the forms, but I really need some time to talk with the doctor before my examination."

"Hold on please..." I waited. "I'll have the doctor's nurse call you back."

I told a nurse about my history hoping she would relay it accurately to the doctor. When I finally got in to see the Dr. Gupta several months later, I was hopeful. The University of Tennessee Medical Center is big. They have an impressive reputation for research, and I was proud that my husband was studying there. I felt positive that they would help me find a solution to my vaginal exasperation.

"So, you have a long history of yeast infection?" a small Indian woman asked over her glasses.

"Yes, but I don't think it is yeast that is causing the problem," I said.

"No? What do you think is the problem?"

"I don't know. I was hoping you would have some ideas?"

"Hmmmm," she thought for a minute. "Have you ever been checked for verms?"

"Verms?" I asked, racking my brain for an STD or an infection in my internet searches. "I don't think so. What is verms?"

"Verms," she said. " You know, the verms?"

"Verms?"

"No, verms!"

"Oh, worms!" I said, "No, I don't think I have been tested for worms. Could that be the problem?"

"It could be," she said. "I think we will do a test for verms." The "verm" test came back negative. Dr. Gupta and I became good friends and still laugh about my "verms." Unfortunately, the "verms" were not my problem.

Next I tried a private practice. I was so desperate at this point that I had begun researching labiectomies. I wanted to remove my inner labia because a lot of the irritation occurred there. Desperate minds make demented decisions. I had simply concluded that if I did not have my labia, it could not cause me pain.

As I walked out in tears from the visit, after telling the doctor he would want his penis removed, too, if it felt like my vagina, a young resident stopped me. She had been in the office for part of the visit but had left before it ended. She held my elbow quickly and said, "Research vaginosis and vulvodynia."

I did. I found an entire culture of women just like me in chat rooms, on the vulvodynia society web page, and on health forums. I was not alone! The problem was, though, not one of them had found a cure.

I went to a specialist who had a theory that women with vaginitis and vaginosis, or vulvodynia suffered from tiny tears in the lining of their vulvas. He treated me with a cream that was successful with patients who had interstitial cystitis. The cream was supposed to heal the tiny tears and provide relief. Thank you for your effort doctor; I know I am not a physician, but your theory did not work for me.

None of my efforts provided any relief. This is the point where so many of the women I talked to for this book remain: stuck and hopeless.

Recommendations
For Vulvodynia Treatments

Treatments for vulvodynia range from the mundane use of antidepressants to invasive surgery. I tried antidepressants, biofeedback, and local anesthetics. I was to the point of considering surgery. I don't know why there was pain and irritation even when I tested negative for yeast. I do know that I relied on lidocaine and Cortisone® cream for years to manage the pain and irritation.

Vulvodynia treatments focus on relieving symptoms. No one treatment works for every woman, and you may find that a combination of treatments works best for you. It may take weeks or even months for treatment to improve your symptoms noticeably. According to the Mayo Clinic, these are the recommended treatments for vulvodynia:

Medications. Tricyclic antidepressants or anticonvulsants may help lessen chronic pain. Antihistamines may reduce itching.

Biofeedback therapy. This therapy can help reduce pain by teaching you how to control specific body responses. The goal of biofeedback is to help you relax to decrease pain sensation. To cope with vulvodynia, biofeedback can teach you to relax your pelvic muscles, which can contract in anticipation of pain and actually cause chronic pain.

Local anesthetics. Medications, such as lidocaine ointment, can provide temporary symptom relief. Your doctor may recommend applying lidocaine 30 minutes before sexual intercourse to reduce your discomfort. If you use lidocaine ointment, your partner also may experience temporary numbness after sexual contact.

Nerve blocks. Women who have long-standing pain that doesn't respond to other treatments may benefit from local injections of nerve blocks.

Pelvic floor therapy. Many women with vulvodynia have problems with the muscles of the pelvic floor, which supports the uterus, bladder, and bowel. Exercises to strengthen those muscles may help relieve vulvodynia pain.

Surgery. In cases in which painful areas can be specifically pinpointed at the hymeneal ring (localized vulvodynia, vulvar vestibulitis), surgery to remove the affected skin and tissue (vestibulectomy) relieves pain in some women.

Amy Stein, author of *Heal Pelvis Pain*, offers useful advice in her book for women who cannot afford to pay for physical therapy.

The thousands of women who participate in vulvodynia support groups have tried all manners of treatments, most with very little relief. Because medicine does not have any definite answers, I want to share what works for the women I talked to. The results varied, but there were some who were completely healed.

I found dozens of women who resolved pH balance issues or healed through diet changes. One woman had no clue how, after seven years of pain, her vulvodynia disappeared.

Several women said a low oxalate diet cured them. Several women said the birth control pill cured them. I talked to women who found relief from surgery and physical therapy. The others said surrender, deep prayer, meditation, and a Buddhist understanding of pain cured them.

I found a woman who said she was healed by a faith healing. A few women found another diagnosis, like pudendal neuralgia, that was treated and then relieved the vulvodynia. Other women did experience relief from a variety of different practices, but did not find a cure.

The quotes that follow are taken from women who responded to my question, "What helps mitigate symptoms?"

"Coconut oil (unrefined organic) moisturizes and relieves itching. Eating organic and using organic healthcare products to reduce the amount of chemicals I come into contact with also helps. I also use meditation and work on practicing self-care/love. It hasn't been easy, but it's a work in progress!"

"The best results for me came from homeopathic treatments. I'm doing much better than when I was first diagnosed."

"Homeopathic treatments and sitz baths with Epson salt or baking soda with essential oils have worked the best for me. I'm still trying out Lyrica (300mg daily), no change with adding that."

"Gabapentin."

"I do the low oxalate diet, sitz baths, ice packs, pain pills, nerve medication and anything else that may help. I try not to make my problem any worse than it already is."

"Baking soda baths, essential oils such as rosemary and lavender oil, ice packs to temporarily to relieve itch and burning."

"I'm currently taking 300 ml of Gabapentin three times a day, and it's helping. I've only had mild irritation, which makes me a lot happier. I'm not in a sexual relationship at moment [sic] so it's hard to tell if it has helped reduce pain during sex. I'm also using hydrocortisone, which helps for a short while, which I used to use before sex, but it was hit and miss on how much it reduced pain."

"Vaginal probiotics - helped with EVERYTHING for 10 days (thought I was on to something)."

"Coconut oil for lube and moisturizing."

"Physical therapy has been a savior for me! I'm seeing a PT who specializes in manual therapy/pelvic floor now."

"I would have to say my Amitripyline has worked the best. I started out working my way up to 120 mgs. I also did physical therapy for six months with biofeedback. Now I'm on 20 mgs of Ami and using coconut oil for moisturizing and lube. I was doing great, but I'm having a bad flare right now."

"Tried every nerve block and InterStim® procedure. Spinal cord stimulator just made my left foot numb. Percocet, Valium, Imipramine, steroid shots, two vestobulectomies [sic], creams, steroids, anal and vaginal botox, valium suppositories, sitz baths, ice packs, gel pillows, heat packs and finally stem cell procedure."

"Cut out coffee, soda, acidic foods, and junk/processed foods. That also helps immensely."

I want to thank these women for sharing their success tips with other women. It is so comforting to find a community of women going through the same thing when an embarrassing disorder rules your life. It is what made me brave enough to put this topic on paper.

Hope for Solutions

Just as I was about to give up, I became pregnant. Mid-way

through our doctoral programs, Mike and I decided it was the perfect time to start a family. We just didn't think it would happen so quickly. Apparently, even though my vagina was broken, my ovaries and everything else worked incredibly well.

We were excited, nervous, and hopeful, and we couldn't stop smiling! Almost immediately, my vagina was fine. My vagina stayed fine throughout the entire nine months of my pregnancy. Is it any wonder we decided to have a second child ten months after the first?

After our first child was born, I mentioned to the attending physician about my vaginal problems. She said, "Use pH cream when you have sex," as she was walking out. pH cream?

"Where do I get it?" I yelled after her.

She poked her head back in the door, "Wal-Mart!"

The pH Cream helped a lot. For a while, I thought I was fixed. The irritation decreased, and the yeast infections diminished. The other thing that happened in my life, although I didn't count it at the time, was the change in my diet and lifestyle that came with babies. I think this might have been as important as the pH cream. I didn't drink, smoke, or eat food that was bad for my babies. I worked out regularly, and I was healthier than I had ever been.

After our second child was born, we moved back to Mississippi to be closer to our families. The vaginal problems came back, along with the stress and unhealthy lifestyle I resumed after Mike started private practice and began working around the clock and calendar. I found myself at home, in a new town, with an infant and a toddler. I was totally overwhelmed. I had somehow earned a doctorate degree but was a total flunky as a stay-at-home mom.

We ate out a lot because I couldn't figure out how to cook meals with two kids who started getting fussy right around dinnertime. I started drinking wine again every night to relax after finally getting the kids in bed. Wine is loaded with sugar.

I attempted to reclaim my autonomy by starting a horribly ill-conceived business that added even more stress to my system. I remember a blur of activity centered around eating fast food, drinking wine, sleeping, changing diapers, and then starting over.

I don't know why I thought adding more kids into a stressful situation was a good idea, but I'm glad we did. Cecelia was born, and the scales tipped. We could no longer manage the stressful, unhealthy life we had created.

Our old life completely fell apart, and we had to build a new one. Thankfully, I was surrounded by an incredible community of friends, moms, and kids who supported our family through this shift. Our own families encouraged us as well.

Our new life is based on healthy living and a family that nourishes each other. We rearranged our priorities, lined up our lives with our values, and stepped out of the rat race. Mike got a partner and went half-time.

After spending three years without a single day off, we took a six-week long vacation. We learned to grow healthy food, make healthy decisions for our kids, and embrace health as a way of life for our whole family.

When Cecelia was almost a year old I met a woman, Nancy, who, ironically, I had met before in Knoxville, although I didn't put it together until much later. She was an original board member of the non-profit Mike and I helped start and a natural health practitioner. We became friends, and I told her about my vagina problems. Nancy changed my life.

At this point, I was willing to try anything to get relief. She said, "It sounds like you have a chronic inflammation and possibly yeast in your body."

I tried not to scream at her, "Believe me, I've taken the probiotic pills and eaten enough yogurt to last a lifetime. It doesn't touch it." In fact, I thought Nancy was a bit "out there." I knew my problems were physical and expected a medical solution.

"I don't mean vaginal yeast," she said. "I mean systemic yeast and chronic inflammation." I had no idea what she was talking about, but I was willing to try anything. Nancy was into fermented foods. In fact, she was crazy about the benefits of fermented foods for human health. She talked on and on about how all cultures preserved foods with methods of fermentation and how those protective bacteria are missing from our diets in modern culture. She was way ahead of all the research you now hear about the microbiome.

She taught me how to make cultured cabbage. Please understand that if you have serious vagina problems, I know you are about to throw this book. Just wait. I started eating fermented cabbage that smelled so bad my kids would run out of the room screaming when I opened a jar. I ate a few bites on blue corn chips every day. After about a week, I started craving it in the afternoons. I probably ate a dozen quart jars worth of cabbage in the first few months.

Then, Nancy taught me how to make kefir. It is a fermented milk product that tastes like buttermilk if you don't add fruit or honey. If you ferment it long enough, it is 99 percent lactose-free. I thought it tasted horrible, but I drank a little every day. You have to understand that after actively seeking out boric acid supplements and trying to have my labia removed, drinking an unpleasant drink was a cakewalk. You can buy kefir at the store, but they add lots of sugar into it.

There are recipes for all sorts of fermented foods online. My favorite books are *Wild Fermentation* by Salvador Katz and *Nourished Kitchen*, by Sally Fallon. Adding fermented foods came after we had significantly cleaned up our lifestyle as a whole. Finding Dr. Terry Wahls *Minding My Mitochondria: How I Overcame Secondary Progressive Multiple Sclerosis and Got Out of My Wheelchair* was a huge motivator.

In six months, my vagina was healed. I do not mean that my vagina was less afflicted. I mean it was healed. Here is the best part: four years later, it still is.

I have gotten two yeast infections in four years. I consider that normal. As soon as I felt them coming on, I upped my fermented food intake and used vaginal probiotics. If I feel any sense of vaginal discomfort, I do the same thing. Gone in several hours. No drugs. No waiting three days. Gone. The vulvodynia, or generalized discomfort from sex, or just irritation from no cause at all, also disappeared. I can't say it strongly enough. I HAVE A NORMAL VAGINA. (Oh, my poor mother.)

Here is what I think is important. A microbiome is the ecological community of commensal, symbiotic, and pathogenic microorganisms that literally share our body space. There are way more protective bacteria in our bodies than harmful ones, or there are supposed to be. Our microbiome is damaged by three main culprits: chemical exposure, food, and infection. Some people have genes that can handle that assault. Others, like myself, do not. Like many women my age, I was not breastfed. Then I contracted one ear infection after another as a child and was treated with untold amounts of antibiotics. Any positive microflora I might have had left were certainly wiped out. Add into that an assault from chemically produced food and food sensitivities, and wham!

Once I removed a lot of the chemical load by changing to a natural diet during pregnancies and added back tons of good microbes to my body through fermented foods, the balance tipped back to normal. It makes sense.

I want to share another success story, because they vary. Tamika wrote, "I went on Nortiptylene to calm my nerves down when I was diagnosed with vulvodynia. I got some relief, but not totally." She does Amy Stein's stretching exercises daily and took physical therapy once a week for three months. She has since backed off the Nortiptylene because of weight gain an started taking Vitamin D, folic acid, and a women's probiotic. She abstained from sex until she thought she had the pain under control.

Amazingly, Tamika reports feeling better since resuming sexual activity. She says she is 90-95 percent well at this time and plans to stop her medication all together soon. She believes the combination of a quick diagnosis, physical therapy, medicine, diet and supplements along with lifestyle changes like changing to cotton undies and organic pads were the key to her quick turn around.

There are common factors among women who have healed from vulvar pain. I spent six months finding out what they are and will set out a protocol based on my conclusions at the end of the chapter. What is disturbing, however, is the wild and wide range of treatments thrown at this disorder and the vastly varying results.

I believe the knowledge about how to remedy this debilitating condition is out there. I think we can say with some confidence what does not work and what does. The problem appears to be a cultural need for a diagnosis and cure from a doctor's office. Unfortunately, this is not where most women are receiving answers. The women I interviewed who were cured found these cures on their own. I will share their practices at the end of this chapter.

Endometriosis

Endometriosis is an often painful disorder affecting one in ten women in which tissue that normally lines the inside of your uterus grows outside your uterus. Endometriosis most commonly involves your ovaries, bowel, or the tissue lining your pelvis. Sometimes, endometrial tissue may spread beyond your pelvic region. I grew up with lots of girls who were ultimately told their horrible periods and later, trouble conceiving, was due to this disorder.

According to the Mayo Clinic, most women report pain associated with their menstrual cycle and note that the pain increases over time. Common signs and symptoms of endometriosis may include: painful periods, pain with intercourse, pain with bowel movements or urination, excessive bleeding, infertility, or other symptoms like fatigue and nausea.

Like so many of the women's ailments discussed in this chapter, the why of endometriosis is not clearly understood. Research suggests it may be hereditary or tied to medical conditions associated with menstrual flow, but that is about all I could find. The treatments are hormone therapy, pain meds, surgery, and assisted reproductive therapies.

There is a new drug on the market called Visanne, which is being promoted by Australian model Syl Freedmon. After suffering from endometriosis for years and undergoing two surgeries with no relief, Syl says this is the answer for her, but it isn't currently available in her home of Australia. "I don't understand why people don't know about it or don't talk about it," she says. "People probably think it's 'icky women's business' and a bit of a taboo topic. It's definitely not cute to talk about."

For a holistic guide to living pain free with endometriosis try *Endometriosis: A Holistic Healing Guide* by Tammy Lorraine Majchrzak. Also, see the Endometriosis Research Center, a non-profit organization with free membership and a wealth of information. I also love the blog *Endometriosis, My Life with You* written by a young girl who is going through all the therapies recommended by her doctor and reporting her progress.

In my conversations with women for this book I heard all kinds of cures. Diet was among the top responses, although what diets varied greatly. Surgery worked for some, but not many. Certain drugs worked, but which drugs varied. Pregnancy was the most consistent answer, ironically. Many women said it was the only cure.

All the women said the pain was debilitating and that they felt isolated and depressed by their chronic condition. I know the feeling! The one thing I know we can do as a culture is to bring these issues right out of the closet and onto the kitchen table. One in ten women is going about her daily life with this thing—the least we can do is say, "You are absolutely not alone." We can listen to each other's stories and share what worked for us. We can support these women while they search for what works for them.

Interstitial Cystitis

Interstitial Cystitis can affect men and women and is also called painful bladder syndrome. People with IC experience discomfort, pressure, burning, pelvic pain, and irritation that ranges in severity. "IC feels like a constant bladder infection with no relief in sight," said a friend of mine who has suffered with IC since having her last child. Some people do experience periods of relief, but others say their symptoms are constant. The theories out there about where it comes from range from a physical abnormality, to allergies, to autoimmune disorders, to heredity. The Mayo Clinic lists physical therapy, oral medications, and nerve therapies among treatments.

Several oral medications may improve the signs and symptoms of interstitial cystitis, according to the Mayo Clinic. Nonsteroidal anti-inflammatory drugs, such as ibuprofen (Advil, Motrin IB, others) or naproxen (Aleve), are used to relieve pain. Tricyclic antidepressants, such as amitriptyline or imipramine (Tofranil), help relax your bladder and block pain. Antihistamines, such as loratadine (Claritin, others), may reduce urinary urgency and frequency and relieve other symptoms.

Pentosan (Elmiron) is approved by the Food and Drug Administration specifically for treating interstitial cystitis. How it works is unknown, but it may restore the inner surface of the bladder, which protects the bladder wall from substances in urine that could irritate it. It may take two to four months before you begin to feel pain relief and up to six months to experience a decrease in urinary frequency.

Certain nerve stimulation techniques include transcutaneous electrical nerve stimulation, which increases blood flow to the bladder, strengthening those muscles, and sacral nerve stimulation. Sacra nerves are a primary link between the spinal cord and nerves in your bladder. Stimulating these nerves may reduce urinary urgency associated with interstitial cystitis.

Bladder distention and medications instilled into the bladder are other forms of treatment. Surgery is also an option, but only as a last resort. Surgeries include figuration to burn off ulcers in the urethra, re-sectioning the bladder, and bladder augmentation to remove damaged portions of the bladder.

One of the most comprehensive websites I found on IC was www.womentowomen.com. It was founded by Marcelle Pick, OB/GYN, NP. Their treatment suggestion page on IC is the most thorough. Possible causes listed include chemicals in urine, mast cell activation, previous bladder damage, and the hormone connection. Recommendations include finding out food triggers, identifying underlying bladder damage causes, balancing hormones, and using anti-inflammatory medicines or supplements, probiotics, physical therapy, and mind-body work.

Polycystic Ovary Syndrome, Ovarian Cysts, Uterine Fibroids, Pelvic Organ Prolapse And Chronic Pelvic Pain

There are a number of other disorders women suffer from. Modern medicine has some effective treatments. I have identified some well received alternative treatment resources as well.

Polycystic Ovary Syndrome is an endocrine disorder where women have enlarged ovaries that contain small collections of fluids. Symptoms include prolonged menstrual periods, excess hair growth, acne, obesity, and painful periods. Causes include excess insulin, low-grade inflammation, and heredity.

Polycystic Ovary Syndrome contributes to many other complications including Type 2 diabetes, depression, high blood pressure, and infertility. BellaOnline.com's infertility editor discussed PCOS and infertility. The article sourced Melissa Diane Smith, a nutritionist, health educator, and author of *Going Against the Grain*. She says 85 percent of her PCOS clients test positive for a sensitivity to gluten. "When these women remove gluten from their diets they often see a marked improvement in their PCOS symptoms."

Ovarian cysts and uterine fibroids are common at various times in most women, but in some individuals, they cause pain and discomfort. Hormone therapy or surgery is usually recommended if the pain does not resolve on its own. There is a lot of writing surrounding diet, hormones, exercise, and natural supplements when it comes to fibroids and cysts. Alternative treatments to these disorders are available in an article by Dr. Tori Hudsgon, N.D. and in books like Dr. Nelson Stringer M.D.'s *Uterine Fibroids: What Every Woman Needs to Know*.

Pelvic Organ Prolapse comes from weakened pelvic floor muscles, usually after childbirth and during menopause. Physical therapy and surgical options are available, but there is a large lawsuit against the transvaginal mesh surgeries done on thousands of women. Hysterectomies are no longer a first line of treatment.

Currently, new surgeries and a vaginal insert are on the rise. *Whole Woman Inc.* at savingthewholewoman.com gives the most honest look at alternative treatments I can find if you are looking for answers outside of surgery. This website is based on the book *Saving the Whole Woman* by RN Christine Anne Kent.

Chronic Pelvic Pain is one of the most misunderstood diagnoses among female disorders. Often associated with past trauma, structural abnormalities, or another disease, Chronic Pelvic Pain has a range of symptoms, including pelvic and abdominal pain or pain during sex, and there has been little success in terms of treatment. Most women who are diagnosed with Chronic Pelvic Pain have no known cause. Hormone treatments, antidepressants, and physical therapy are among the common treatments.

I equate Chronic Pelvic Pain to vulvodynia of the pelvis. There are dozens of treatments, mainstream and alternative, that help manage pain symptoms, but the cures I found were very similar to the cures for vulvodynia (see next section). I recommend *Heal Pelvic Pain: The Proven Stretching, Strengthening, and Nutrition Program for Relieving Pain, Incontinence, & I.B.S, and Other Symptoms Without Surgery* by Amy Stein for a detailed overview.

Conclusion and Recommendations

I am not a scientist. I am not a doctor, but at one point, I was a qualitative researcher in educational administration. Qualitative researchers do not use hard numbers to draw conclusions. They do not use double-blind studies or correlation quotients. Qualitative researchers use something called triangulation. If enough stories, observations, or data point to the same theme, you can assume it has some validity.

I have talked to hundreds of women about the disorders covered in this chapter. I have watched dozens of You Tube videos and webinars from people who say they have healed. This is what I believe these testimonies point to: vulvodynia and many, maybe even all, of the disorders covered above function like autoimmune disorders. Talking with Dr. Terry Wahls for the Preface of this book confirmed this conclusion. I read recently that all disease is caused by an inflammatory response of one kind or another. Whatever the cause, something makes the body attack itself. Something makes these disorders run in groups. No one has just vulvodynia. They also have irritable bowel syndrome, depression, reflux, interstitial cystitis, PMS, or other inflammatory disorders. Similar to other autoimmune disorders, Western medicine has very few answers.

Autoimmune disorders are on the rise across the board. Modern diet and lifestyle are two of the main culprits. The good news is that individual people do have solutions. When I take out just the responses from women who say they are completely healed, not 80 percent, or 90 percent, or even 95 percent healed, but 100 percent well, I get a pretty clear protocol.

The problem is not that we don't have a protocol for healing these disorders. The problem is that women have been culturally trained to look for solutions only in doctor's offices. We want a medication or a procedure. We want a medical solution that comes in a bottle or an operating room. We want to be able to be well and keep our artificial sweeteners and coffee beverages. Unfortunately, I only found a handful of women who were cured this way. The majority of women who were totally healed from any of the disorders covered in this chapter did it one of two ways: major systemic health overhaul or mind/body/spirit work.

These were not the answers I wanted to present to desperate women. I wanted to be able to share success stories that were easily attainable. However, the truth is that you have to work hard to regain health, and you have to give up some of the things you love in order to be well.

I changed my diet and lifestyle dramatically, and I have to continue that lifestyle to keep the results. There are really good case studies on hundreds of women who have healed themselves the same way. While I suspected there would be a lot of women who healed from diet and lifestyle changes, I did not predict the number of women I would find who healed completely from mind-body or spiritual work.

I found enough of them that I feel compelled to include them and I am changing my own attitudes toward these practices and their implications for health.

Based on my search for healed women, these are the factors most often held in common:

1) Rule out a physical cause and boost your overall immune system. Some women did find underlying, identifiable causes for vulvodynia. Get a thorough work up done, including labs and a physical exam. Look for things that might not be directly related but that can affect overall health. Do the work to boost your immune system.

2) Go on an elimination diet to find out what foods your body reacts to. This is not the same for everyone. You have to find out what foods irritate you. Follow a plan like the GAPs diet or the Clean Gut Diet. Make this step your priority. It is the hardest but most important step. If you cannot find out what foods cause inflammatory responses in your body, you cannot get well. The seven most common food triggers are: gluten, dairy, nuts, sugar, sugar substitutes, eggs, soy, caffeine, and shellfish. Eat simple, few ingredient meals until you know what you can tolerate. Keep a food journal. When you can, eat clean food: organic, grass-fed, and naturally grown. Grow a garden or find a farmer's market to make healthy food financially viable.

3) Cut out sugar. Just cut it. There is no health benefit on earth to sugar. If you want to be well, cut sugar out of your diet for one month and see how you feel. I sweeten almost everything with honey in our house. If you cannot conceive of going a month without sugar, you have just proven how utterly addicted you are to a harmful and inflammatory substance. I know this is the hardest one, but is it harder than feeling awful all the time?

4) Balance your body's pH. Buy test strips and urinate on them regularly. Cut out foods that raise pH, and add in foods that lower it. Read books on the science behind balancing your pH. There is a lot of information out there. Many women who cured themselves through diet and lifestyle said their pH was now normal. Mine is now normal, although I did not follow a low oxalate diet. I believe it normalized by cleaning up my whole system.

5) Get rid of systemic yeast. Seal and heal the gut by eliminating triggers and adding fermented foods. Historically, every culture on earth ate fermented foods as part of their normal diets. Modern food preservation systems

remove the need for fermentation resulting in a modern culture deficient in good gut bacteria. Flood yourself with probiotic rich foods, not the pills. Fermented foods need to become part of our modern, typical diet to rid the body of systemic yeast and replace bad bacteria with good bacteria throughout the gut lining. Buy the book *The Art of Fermentation* by Sandor Katz and get started making fermented food. Adding fermented foods was *the* cornerstone to my healing.

6) Implement the Wahls Protocol. Increase your consumption of vegetables significantly. It is so simple: If we don't feed our cells what they need to function correctly, they won't. Our DNA will determine where the weak spots in our immune system are and we will begin to demonstrate signs of illness and disease in those areas.

7) Learn about the mind-body connection and how it impacts wellness. The one thing every healed person did was manage stress proactively, exercise, and meditate. Most of them promoted gentle exercise like yoga or walking, but all of them subscribed to meditation or prayer.

8) Physical Therapy helped hundreds of women who had vaginal tightening or spasms. If you can't afford to go to a physical therapist, there are affordable books and videos that teach these techniques. Many women had success doing the exercises at home on a regular basis.

9) Do not cheat until you are well, but don't give up if you do fall off the wagon. This is a systemic overhaul—a lifestyle change. Until you are ready to take on health as a whole lifestyle, wellness will evade you. There is no pill or quick fix. Every healed person said it took time, persistence, and serious commitment. Several said they tried half-heartedly to change their diet with no success until they gave their health a major overhaul. Some said once they achieved wellness they were able to cheat a little, but not until they had been

well for a long time. Everyone who achieved wellness said it no longer felt hard to live a healthy lifestyle.

10) Take high quality vitamins and supplements. Some autoimmune disorders respond really well to supplements if there is a vitamin or mineral deficiency. You can get most of these through foods, but in the beginning, in order to get your levels up, you may want to take several supplements. Vitamins D, C, B, and Fish Oil are some of the most important. There are dozens of herbs that you can incorporate into your diet through teas that are high in vitamins and minerals your body needs. If you are unsure which are the most important, have a Metabolic Panel run and begin with a good multi-vitamin. There are dozens of books on autoimmune disorders and supplements. Start reading!

There is a fearless woman named Laura Lerhaupt who has written an excellent e-book on healing vulvodynia. It is a guide to healing you can follow step by step. She will send it to you at no charge if you email her at bewelllaural@gmail.com. Her protocol is a well-written guide to reclaiming health for women's issues and mirrors protocols I have seen for Endometriosis, Interstitial Cystitis, Cyst and Fibroid Treatments, but it is much more in depth than anything available on the market.

If you are interested in learning about the mind-body work many women attribute to their healing, there are several books listed in the resources section. The landmark work is *The Mindbody Prescription: Healing the Body, Healing the Pain* by John E. Sarno M.D. Lorraine Faehndrich owns *Radiant Life Designs* http://radiantlifedesigns and is the only health coach I have found who deals specifically with vaginal and pelvic pain relief, although there are others who deal with pain in general. I took her online seminar last year and she knows her stuff.

Finally, prayer and meditation played a huge role in many women's healing. Almost every woman who attributed their health to diet and lifestyle changes included prayer and meditation in their weekly, if not daily, regimens. I spoke with several women who believe the single factor that healed them was faith. I could not begin to list resources for developing a spiritual life, but if you are serious about becoming well, I would not discount it as an important part of healing and wellness.

What I want to emphasize is hope. There are lots of women out there who are healed. There are some definite patterns to what they did to heal. If you are among the women whose lives are completely ruled by vulvar, uterine, or bladder pain, you can get better. Be fearless and do the work. Life is so sweet on the other side.

Section 3

The Mother

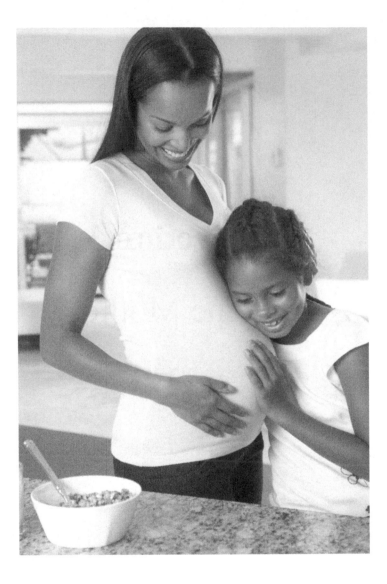

SECTION FOREWORD

"We are the girls with anxiety disorders, filled appointment books, five-year plans. We take ourselves very, very seriously. We are the peacemakers, the do-gooders, the givers, the savers. We are on time, overly prepared, well read, and witty, intellectually curious, always moving... We pride ourselves on getting as little sleep as possible and thrive on self-deprivation. We drink coffee, a lot of it. We are on birth control, Prozac, and multivitamins... We are relentless, judgmental with ourselves, and forgiving to others... We are the daughters of the feminists who said, "You can be anything," and we heard, "You have to be everything.""

—**Courtney Martin**

Daughters of Feminists

Our grandmothers and mothers freed my generation of women. They gave us more choices than women have ever been afforded. I want to thank these incredibly bright, talented, determined, and strong women. The possibilities of our lives rest on their efforts.

I am afraid what we have done since the ceiling was reached is not entirely inspiring. Just like when teenagers move out of the house for the first time into the freedom of adulthood there is a lot of learning to do. There are so many mistakes to make. So many ways we could use, abuse, ignore, or thrive in our freedom. So many ways we could waste it or make it something awesome.

Post-feminism is intriguing to me, but I believe its success is balanced precariously. I never thought that in my lifetime I would hear contemporaries saying things such as, "The husband is the head of the household." I hear it all the time now. Neo-conservative family values are currently popular in America. They are thriving in churches and on American Family Radio programs.

Well-educated women are writing books on the subject. I keep

127

asking myself what these women are trying to achieve when they take this stance. What line are they drawing, and why are they drawing it? Why are women running from the equality our grandmothers and mothers fought for? Why are we not equally terrified of our own fundamentalist shift as we are of the spread of fundamentalism abroad?

In my lifetime, Iran has gone from a place where women had the right to vote (it was granted by the Shah in 1962) to a place where women can be stoned to death for owning a mobile phone, according to the *Independent*. I am convinced that the backlash against women's independence is a result of our insecurity about what to do with it and the realization that the world we gained access to is not everything we thought it would be. Freedom, independence, and autonomy are all words with two sides.

On one side they are empowering; on the other, they are lonely, frustrating, and frightening. Post-feminists recognize the double-edged-sword feminism acquired for us, and a lot of women have looked around and summed up the situation as overrated, false, or just plain scary.

We realize that we gained access to a system that is fundamentally broken. Greater opportunities for women in the workplace inducted us into the same bankrupt, stress-ridden, rat race where powerful men reside, and we want to hand it back.

There is another way, a third way, to achieve independence. This way is an evolving feminism where women don't try to be like men; instead, we hold secure to the power we have as women. We thought we wanted to enter and own a piece of men's worlds, but what I think we are beginning to recognize is a need for access to a better world where women's strengths are respected in their own right. Post-feminists understand that being a woman is an incredible gift when we live in a society where it is upheld as a valuable and equally important role. We need more feminists in a world where political leaders make decisions by thumping their chests. We need more feminists in a world where social policy devalues caregivers.

The lowest paid positions in our culture are those most directly tied to hands-on care. This is a time for females to step up in powerful ways. "Mothering" may be the most commanding role available to women, after all, but only if we claim it as the vital position it is, rather than resigning ourselves to the role because there are no other options.

This section of the book deals with issues very central to feminism: birth control, fertility, pregnancy, and caregiving. The Mother archetype does not require having given physical birth. Qualities of The Mother can be embodied by all people. Caring, demonstrating compassion, showing strength, nourishing ourselves and others, and valuing relationships are among these qualities. They are not soft attributes. Picture those pioneer women; were they soft? Caring is among the hardest work known to humans and needs to be valued accordingly.

I believe that women and men are figuring out how to creatively deal with gender roles in new and positive ways. I also believe that it is messy business. Change is always messy. I am a woman with a doctorate degree who stays home with my children. I argue with myself about my identity daily. I try not to argue with my friends over differing values related to women's choices and motherhood. However, I do *not* abide radio talk-shows drenched in false religiosity that try to shove women back into small boxes with jokes and slick tongues. Listen to the jokes carefully with attention to inference and intent. They are not funny and they are not Christian, but they are all over the airwaves as I drive my kids to school.

Rules and well-defined positions are comfortable in their inability to surprise us, make us unsure of ourselves, or push us to the edge of our comfort zones. They are also dangerous. Pick any chapter out of history, and observe what happens when people are driven by fear rather than confidence. Don't be scared. We can figure this out. What our mothers and grandmothers fought for, and what our fathers and grandfathers supported because they knew it was right, was the freedom to make choices. They campaigned to make sure being born a female was an asset, not a curse. Working, staying at home, using birth control, using natural family planning, natural childbirth, scheduled c-sections, breastfeeding, bottle-feeding, breadwinning, all of it comes down to the possibility of choices that did not exist in previous generations, and will not continue to exist if we abandon these victories out of fear.

What we need to focus our energy on is a different set of questions altogether. What choices make us healthier people? What choices most effectively support our children? What choices are in the best interest of our communities, overall? How do the effects of our choices ripple out into the world, and what kind of world do we want for our children? They are not easy questions, but they are vital. I want all parties at the table, on equal footing, shaping the future for my kids.

Chapter 7

Family Planning

"The Church's stand on birth control is the most absolutely spiritual of all her stands and with all of us being materialists at heart, there is little wonder that it causes unease. I wish various fathers would quit trying to defend it by saying that the world can support 40 billion. I will rejoice the day when they say: This is right whether we all rot on top of each other or not, dear children, as we certainly may. Either practice restraint or be prepared for crowding... "—**Flannery O'Connor**

"Woman must have her freedom, the fundamental freedom of choosing whether or not she will be a mother and how many children she will have. Regardless of what man's attitude may be, that problem is hers — and before it can be his, it is hers alone. She goes through the vale of death alone, each time a babe is born. As it is the right neither of man nor the state to coerce her into this ordeal, so it is her right to decide whether she will endure it"
—**Margaret Sanger**

I must be a fool to take on birth control in writing. I am certainly going to turn someone off. It is not my goal to make people angry, but to provide information on the subject that cannot be as easily found. Thankfully, although I wouldn't do it again, I have had tubal ligation and no longer have to deal with this issue myself, but may soon have to face it with my children. I want to open up the dialogue just a bit wider than it was in my reproductive time.

At one time in my life, I felt like birth control was a marker of an educated society, possibly *the* marker. Over time, I have mellowed some on my stance. Issues surrounding birth control are often divided into liberal and conservative camps, but those labels are unhelpful and distracting at this time in our history. I have known self-affirmed liberal folks who believe that practicing natural cycle awareness (formerly called the rhythm method) is effective. I have met self-affirmed libertarians who want to take dramatic measures to reduce the world's population.

In my experience, you cannot put people into camps based on their beliefs about birth control. How many Catholics do you know who love both the Pope and the Pill? How many anti-abortion advocates do you know who wouldn't mind aborting entire nations of Muslims? These beliefs and values are rarely based on what makes sense and center more on our biggest fears or most passionate ideals.

I would like to take another look in this chapter at how our personal beliefs and choices, which are shaped by our cultural context, impact family planning. I also want to look critically at our current options for birth control.

I am at a golden point of life. I am between the age when I no longer have to worry about becoming pregnant myself and the age when I will have to worry about my kids getting pregnant or getting someone else's kid pregnant. I always welcome real feedback from parents who feel like they have good input on how to deal with reproductive-aged children.

I want to look at birth control as it exists today. What are the options our there? What are the pros and cons of these options? What long-term impact does the birth control method, or lack of one, that we use, have on us? What should we teach our kids?

When I began looking up the most recent information on birth control, I went to the gurus at Planned Parenthood. I also researched some of the largest religious organizations' publications and some of the most influential natural living organizations. I also looked at what cultures that are not highly influenced by religious values say about birth control. This chapter is based on a synthesis of all my findings from these combined resources.

Moral and Religious Arguments For and Against Birth Control

Birth control, among Americans, is often attached to some form of religious belief. I have been fascinated by conversations on sexuality with a friend from Japan, a culture very uninfluenced by religions. I wanted to know how cultures that are not dominated by a religious culture deal with birth control. The answers vary widely.

Dutch culture, where two-thirds of the parents surveyed said they allowed boyfriends and girlfriends to have sleep-overs, have the lowest teen pregnancy rates—the Dutch actually place a high value on teenage love, according to T. Rios in *Teen Pregnancy Rates Around the World.*

While they don't appear to discourage sexual activity at all, they do emphasize loving, respectful relationships. They promote the "Double Dutch" method of using the birth control pill combined with a male condom. Japanese culture places a value on high moral standards and not bringing shame to the family; although these standards are changing as they are everywhere. Japanese teens tend to wait longer before having sex, and the stigma for teen moms continues to dictate behavior, according to Knoji.com. Teen pregnancy in Japan is among the lowest in the world.

On the other end of the spectrum, China rigidly legislates birth control to reduce population growth. Overpopulation is a very critical issue worldwide. By 2025, the global population is expected to reach eight billion. According to Worldwatch.org, India and several countries in Africa lead the world in growth. Within the next few decades, the east African nation of Uganda is likely to have the highest population growth in the world. According to Carl Haub, a demographer at Population Reference Bureau, the Ugandan government's lack of commitment to family planning is the main

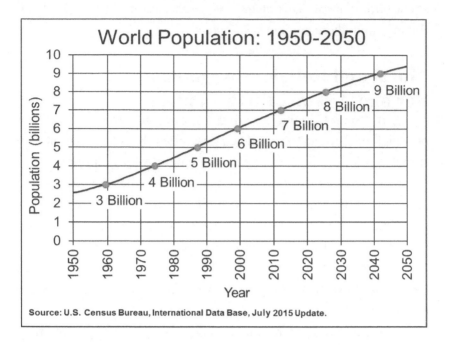

World Population: 1950-2050

Source: U.S. Census Bureau, International Data Base, July 2015 Update.

reason for the country's extraordinary population growth.

Some of the opposition's main moral arguments against birth control are founded on the fear of imperialism or misuse of power, as seen in China, and on the premise that birth control increases sexual leniency and social and health problems.

Proponents of birth control believe that it is evolutionarily relevant and necessary and that birth control solves many of society's social, health, and gender problems.

Moral Arguments Surrounding Birth Control

There are three main moral arguments against the use of birth control. The first is based on the premise that controlling the natural process of fertility and birth is inherently wrong. This argument sees all birth control as unnatural, anti-life, and abortive.

People who follow this vein of thinking believe that it is

134

immoral to separate sex from reproduction. The second moral argument asserts that using birth control brings negative consequences like health risks, cultural decline, and mass population control. Writings promoting this argument voice concern about birth control preventing the birth of a person who might ultimately help humanity. The third moral argument asserts that birth control encourages immoral behavior.

When sex is no longer tied to the consequences of producing life, the increased likelihood of sex outside of marriage, affairs, and sexual deviance increases, according to this argument.

The moral arguments in favor of birth control assert there is no reason birth control should be viewed as morally wrong. Additionally, these advocates assert that the benefits of using birth control far outweigh any other argument.

Proponents argue for "procreative liberty," the freedom birth control allows humans to attain their life goals, health benefits, family benefits, benefits for women, and population benefits. Their arguments often directly tie women's health, economic, and gender status to the availability of birth control, according to BBC Ethics Guide.

Religious Views on Birth Control

Most religious views on birth control do not appear to come directly from religious texts; rather, they are conceived from interpretations of scripture's views on procreation. Judeo-Christian, Muslim, and Mormon beliefs about contraception are based on these three premises: being fruitful and multiplying, not interfering with the will of God, and having sex only within the bounds of marriage.

Buddhist views on contraception come from the understanding that all life is sacred. Methods that prevent conception are acceptable. Hindu views on birth control appear to be related to two factors: duty to raise families and overpopulation. In all religions, the spectrum of individuals' views on birth control is wide. There are liberal and conservative interpretations of the use of birth control among all faiths. Most religions I looked at had active camps on both sides of the issue.

American religious views create conflicting behaviors concerning birth control. Our Puritan roots make birth control an off-limits subject for families and schools, but our spirit of independence drives a strong desire for family planning. Our religious roots may influence our behaviors surrounding the use and acceptance of and the education about birth control more than we realize. Balancing religious beliefs, updated science, and women's health is tricky business, but it is important to recognize the contexts that drive our behaviors.

Methods of Birth Control

I will not recount each form of available birth control. Planned Parenthood has an excellent website on every mode of available birth control and an objective list of the benefits and drawbacks. For a detailed look at all birth control options, I found no better site, and I recommend reading the information they provide. As I was reading each one, I kept thinking, *Why did I never know this?*

I am quite sure I never once read the side effect warnings on any of the half-dozen methods I used in my lifetime. Why not? Did I simply take my friends' words for it? Did I accept that if my doctor would prescribe it, it must be okay? Did I fog over when the lawsuit commercials came on TV or when hearing the humorously long list of possible side effects? Where was I when I made these important decisions that could have had a lasting impact on my health or my family? Why didn't I pay more attention to the decisions that dictated whether or not we brought another member of our family into the world?

There are now dozens of forms of birth control available to women and a few to men. New forms emerge at a staggeringly fast pace. I urge you to become educated on the positive and negative

136

consequences of birth control methods.

I wonder if I would have chosen differently had I done my own research. I wonder what I will think are acceptable risk factors for my daughter. I wonder what health implications medicine will identify in the future. I want us to make our own educated decisions about reproductive health, rather than handing our bodies blindly over to drug companies and government agencies.

Abstinence and Waiting

Abstinence means refraining from sexual intercourse. That is pretty obvious. However, Planned Parenthood's definition includes a distinction between abstinence and celibacy.

People have varying opinions about abstinence. For some abstinence is defined as not having vaginal intercourse. One may be "abstinent" and enjoy other kinds of sex play that don't lead to pregnancy. This is sometimes called "outercourse."

Planned Parenthood also provides suggestions for remaining abstinent when you are in a relationship and advice on how to talk to your partners. Abstinence is listed as the most effective birth control for preventing pregnancy and sexually transmitted diseases.

As addressed in Section 1, fifty percent of young people in the United States are sexually active. However, I do want to address the other fifty percent who are not. These young people are practicing abstinence, and most of them say a religious belief is their reason. According to *Waiting Till Marriage*, one in five people in highly religious organizations wait until marriage to have sex, which is higher than the average of one in thirty among general populations.

Christianity Today is one of the most frequented websites among Christian teens. According to an article entitled "10 Ways to Practice Purity" there are four ideas such teens are encouraged to adhere to. First, they place sex into a larger context of faith. Second, they recognize the reality that refraining from sex when you are in love is hard! Third, they give practical tips on how to remain abstinent. And fourth, they acknowledge that it is human nature to screw up.

Compare the *Christianity Today* article with an article from *Muslim Matters* titled "Sexual Activities Beyond the Norm: What Should We Teach Our Teens." It achieves similar goals of contextualizing sexual activity among unmarried youth, providing practical advice, and acknowledging human nature. The author concludes: "We must keep in mind that our children will slip. This is as long as it is a minor issue, like sexual thoughts or masturbation (major issues like love affairs will have to be dealt with differently). Remind them of fighting their temptations with *du'ā'* and *istighfaar.* Help them fight the *fitnah.* Encourage them to pray *qiyam'l-layl.* Provide them with distractions. Rid them of all the means of falling into sin. Though, be very careful and wise. Do not scare them away by being too tough on them. Remember, they are human beings, and as long as they feel remorse and repent to Allāh, you will have to allow them room to sin a little."

The practice of abstinence is not only based on religious beliefs. Adults of all creeds often subscribe to abstinence for periods of time. Many say fear of disease or causing pregnancy is their reason for remaining abstinent.

Others do so for psychological healing. People may practice abstinence at varying times in their lives for varying reasons.

Synthetic Hormones

I want to talk for a minute about the Pill. At the root of the sexual revolution was the availability of synthetic hormones. The Pill and its later cousins (implants, patches, shots, etc.) appeared at the exact time when social morality about sexuality was undergoing big changes during the sexual revolution.

A generation of women was suddenly freed from fear of an unwanted pregnancy. While many women swear by their method of synthetic hormones, the drawbacks are beginning to surface. In a web log entry, "That Naughty Little Pill," Kelly Brogan, M.D. writes emphatically about her transformation from believing the Pill was a woman's right to considering the "tacit permissiveness toward reckless unprotected sex, the wholesale delegation of contraception to the female counterpart, and the fundamental divorce of a woman from the very feedback systems that fire up her reproductive age vitality."

Brogan began to question biochemical concerns surrounding the pill as well. She wondered how many women had accurate information about the risks of thromboembolism, hypertension, cerebrovascular events, gallstones, and cancer. She also began doing her own research on how the Pill influences sex hormones, thyroid hormones, and adrenal hormones. She writes:

> **When patients come to me with complaints of low libido, low or flat mood, weight gain, hair loss, and cloudy thinking, one of my first questions is, "Are you on the Pill?" When they come complaining about premenstrual irritability, insomnia, tearfulness, bloating, and breast tenderness, requesting that I sanction beginning a course of oral contraceptives and perhaps an antidepressant, the one-size-fits-all-cure-all of psychiatrists and gynecologists nationwide, my first comment is "There's a better way."**

It seems like every day I am hearing of a new undesirable complication from The Pill. I think the conversation about why we accept big trade-offs for birth control is well overdue. Thankfully, there are some new options out there.

While the rhythm method was once relegated to the ultra-religious or the ultra-natural, technology may have made this a viable option for everyone. What other possibilities are out there? What conversations do we need to have about birth control and the real tradeoffs?

New Options

There is one form of birth control not covered under Planned Parenthood. It has been receiving a lot of attention lately from advocates like Dr. Kelly Brogan, so I wanted to include it. It is a digital technology that determines whether or not you are ovulating and is 99 percent effective in preventing pregnancy when used correctly. I found reviews provided by Lady Comp® and Pearly®, the two trademark brands of these devices, but I hold a healthy skepticism of distributor-produced reviews. I found a personal review on evolvingwellness.com which I consider the most helpful:

> **In a nut shell, I LOVE Pearly—and, today, cannot imagine my life without it! I really cannot say enough about it. My only regret is that I did not find out about Pearly sooner, hence one of the reasons why I am so passionate to spread more awareness about this unit. It is not a cheap device, I guess one could say, about $300, but I have to tell you, it is one of the best $300 I ever spent. And for the reliability, ease of use and sophistication of this product, it is a very fair price in my opinion. Using Pearly is so easy, so completely natural and I never have to worry about an unwanted or unexpected pregnancy.**

It appears technology has gotten the rhythm method down to a science. Women who reviewed the product said the only difficult part was remembering to take a reading each morning, at first, but said within a few weeks it became routine.

The device shows a red (do not have sex), yellow (proceed with caution), or green (go ahead) symbol based on your waking body temperature. It becomes more accurate over time showing fewer yellow days. This technology is also helpful for women who are trying to conceive.

Sterilization

Sterilization is where many of us in Western culture end up. For me, it was a relief. According to the NIH, female or male sterilization is the most common contraceptive method utilized by couples in the United States, with 36 percent of fertile women using contraception employing this method. According to the National Survey of Family Growth (2002), 10.3 million women (27 percent) rely on female sterilization for birth control, whereas 3.5 million women (9.2 percent) rely on vasectomy in their partners for contraception.

For others, the decision is filled with regret or complications. The long-term effects of hysterectomies are something millions of women had to live through before doctors began to take a closer look. Thankfully, tying tubes is a much easier procedure than it used to be, and there are several methods to discuss with your doctor.

Vasectomies for men have also improved. There are minimally invasive procedures now that are supposedly less painful. There is some controversy about prostate cancer as a result of vasectomies, although the evidence is inconclusive.

Like so many birth control options, sterilization has only been around for a short time in the span of our human experience. As our population explodes, and as controlling childbirth becomes a way of life, sterilization has become commonplace. We do not typically wind our childbearing years down naturally in Western cultures. We choose when they will end. I make no moral judgments about sterilization, but I do note how far we have come from our natural rhythm of procreation.

A Birth Control Story

For Marta, birth control was always a tricky issue. The Pill or any other hormonal treatments tended to drive her to near insanity. She cried constantly, became irrational and generally felt miserable. The ease with which many other women found contentment with the Pill or other hormonal birth control eluded her.

After giving birth to two children, she tried a hormone-free IUD. After about a week, she experienced painful cramps and realized she couldn't find the string attached to the device. She went to a physician and he told her that her body had sucked the device up into the uterus and he could not get it out. She had to undergo surgery to have it removed. They showed her the device after they removed it and it was all crunched up as if her uterus had tried to squish it.

Next she tried a diaphragm and had some success. Condoms irritated her. When she and her husband decided to have another child they realized it was time for something permanent. She assumed her husband would have a vasectomy, but before they could discuss it her doctor told her that since she would be opened up anyway during the C-section, it would be a good time for him to tie her tubes at the same time.

It made sense to her, but after the procedure she developed a stinging, burning pain in her lower abdomen that didn't occur with the other C-section. She is bitter about that to this day.

Marta's case was an example of should have, could have, would have. Based on my research, if I were concerned about birth control, I would most likely try one of the new non-hormonal, non-invasive methods such as Pearly.

What I hope we will do as a culture is to begin to take a long view of health and wellness. I hope we will begin to look at our bodies as parts of a whole. Is a uterus as disposable as a wisdom tooth? Apparently not. Let's get these topics on the agenda.

Chapter 8
Fertility & Infertility

So now I just assume that it won't work, and that if it does work, I'll lose it anyway. This is meant to protect me, although it doesn't, because somehow the hope sneakily finds its way in. I'm never aware of the hope until it's gone, whooshed away like a rug pulled from under my feet, each time I hear another "I'm sorry."
—**Liane Moriarty**

For many women, myself included, becoming pregnant, or trying to become pregnant, is the first time we really begin to take our health seriously. There is something hopeful about this.

While we may not be vigilant in caring for our own health, nature tends to kick in when we start thinking about taking care of the health of a child.

Part of the premise of this book is to extend that instinct to care for our young children well into their adolescence, but it starts with the very idea of new life.

I do not presume that all pregnancies are happy or wanted, and I cannot say if the instinct to start caring for yourself while carrying a child applies to all pregnancies. Most likely it doesn't. But I do believe it is a good time to reach women with new information. When you are in the completely vulnerable spot of carrying an alien life inside your body for the first time, just about anything seems possible.

I also want to address the growing epidemic of infertility. The heartbreaking inability to conceive is rampant in our culture. Women are waiting longer to have children, which significantly contributes to the rise in infertility, but there are so many other factors at play here. There is an entire medical machine built around fertility that did not exist thirty years ago. Women are subjecting their bodies and finances to the latest trials in order to conceive. I lived through this process with one of my dearest friends, and I know the mental and physical agony over conception is all-consuming.

Some of the issues we need to begin discussing surrounding fertility include cultural expectations, emotionally supporting women who experience infertility, and environmental causes.

Cultural Expectations

Cultural expectations surrounding gender roles have shifted enormously in the last two generations of Western culture. We no longer only give our little girls dolls and our little boys trucks. We are much more accepting of role crossing and gender fluidity for our young people. We want our children to grow up and have opportunities to care for the family, whether they are boys or girls, and to succeed in the world regardless of gender. What I think has not changed is the expectation that women should have and want a child.

I am sure part of our expectation for women to have children is our biological need to procreate our species, but, culturally, what makes it so hard for us to accept childless families? What makes it so hard for childless women to accept their lives as whole or complete? Is it because we live apart from extended families? Historically, would a childless aunt have been an asset to the family as a whole, an integral set of much valued hands, a beloved parent-figure to nieces and nephews? Would life without children seem strange or undesirable in a different cultural context?

I do not have answers, but I do know the enormous pressure women are under, from themselves and from our society, to have a baby in order to feel complete. What does that mean for those of us who cannot or do not want to have a child? What does it mean for those of us who have children but do not feel "maternal?" Is there a way we can bring all women into the fold as "Mothers" in a larger sense? I want to look at the Mother archetype in this chapter and address some of these questions.

Fertility & Infertility

A woman is most fertile between the ages of 20 and 24, exactly the ages most women in Western culture do not want to become pregnant. Our fertility begins to decline at age 27, the age many college-educated women begin thinking about having babies. A more drastic decline in fertility begins at age 35. A healthy thirty-year-old woman has a 20 percent chance of conceiving each month, compared with a 5 percent chance each month by women in their mid-forties, according to R. Gurevich in "7 Things Every Woman Needs To Know About Fertility."

The overall rise in infertility in women of all childbearing age is staggering. According to the CDC's National Survey of Family Growth, the number of women 24 years old and younger who reported trouble conceiving or maintaining a pregnancy has almost doubled in the past two decades. Moreover, 44 percent of women signing up for reproductive assistance now are under 35.

Eleven percent of all women ages 15 to 44, and 12 percent of married women in that age group, have impaired fecundity. Twelve percent of men aged 25 to 44 in 2006–2010 reported some type of infertility. Increasing rates of infertility appear to have reached a plateau as of 2002.

Information on boosting fertility is overwhelming. Maintaining a healthy weight, improving your diet, taking vitamins, incorporating exercise into your life, and improving overall health are the first line suggestions for men and women. Smoking and excess heat significantly reduce sperm count in males. Yet, even when they make these lifestyle changes, many couples continue to struggle to find solutions to infertility.

Fertility clinics abound today, and they target infertility in several ways. If an ovulatory problem is suspected, women may take medications such as Clomiphene, which stimulates the ovaries to release eggs, or Metformin, which is used to treat polycystic ovary syndrome. Unexplained infertility is often treated with Clomiphene, insemination, or hormone injections. If the fallopian tubes are blocked, treatment may include tubal surgery. If mild to moderate endometriosis seems to be the main reason for infertility, treatment may include laparoscopic surgery to remove endometrial tissue growth.

Unlike the simpler process of artificial insemination, in vitro fertilization (IVF) involves combining eggs and sperm outside the body in a laboratory. Once an embryo or embryos form, they are then placed in the uterus. IVF is a complex and expensive procedure, costing between $10,000 and $15,000 for each cycle. Only about 5 percent of couples with infertility seek it out. However, since its introduction in the U.S. in 1981, IVF and other similar techniques have resulted in more than 200,000 babies, according to the National Survey of Family Growth.

There are many success stories from women who undergo fertility treatment and end up giving birth to healthy babies, but the physical toll it takes on women is considerable. The emotional and financial toll these treatments take on families is significant as well.

The following quote was taken from the BBC's series *IVF Hope and Despair:* "I don't know which is worse, having fertility treatment or just sitting around waiting to have it along with that awful feeling that your life is going nowhere. Yet everyone around you seems to be having babies, whether they want them or not. I have been through this awful period of waiting for my life to start for nearly nine years now, and it's shocking to feel as if my life has been on hold for that long."

"On hold" is how many women described trying to get pregnant. I asked my friend Susan, who struggled to have a baby for years, to describe her experience. She was hesitant, then said, "It sucks, but it is so worth it." She wrote:

My husband and I tried for over a year to get pregnant. Finally, we agreed to seek out fertility assistance. We tried Clomid for several months with no success (I was told Lupron was the devil's drug—something you take later, but for me, Clomid was the devil's drug—I was an emotional roller coaster, mood swings, sweating, not feeling at all like myself). I charted my temperatures month after month, and it showed that I was not ovulating, which later was found not to be true. Next, we began IUI treatments along with stronger medications to help build all my hormone levels. After three failed IUI treatments, we moved on to the "big one," IVF treatments.

I can't even begin to tell you how frustrating and emotionally draining those three years were. I once read that the grief you experience going through fertility treatments is very similar to that of cancer patients. I am not saying I would ever trade infertility for cancer. I am just saying that it was something that I thought of every single day. It seemed like every day a friend or coworker was getting pregnant and I was not. I always had 28 day cycles and no other serious health complications. I even rarely got sick. But here I was at 33 years old and desperate to have my own biological child.

After 2 1/2 years of trying, my husband and I were told we should try IVF, and we were ready! I produced too few eggs for my age, and once they formed as embryos, they "fell apart." I believe I had 10 eggs and after five days, there were only two left. They categorized them as a B and C egg. An A level egg is the best type of egg, B is ok, and they only put C in if needed because they don't usually "work." They implanted the two eggs and I received a call after the pregnancy test a few days later saying I was not pregnant. I was devastated. I just cried and cried, feeling hopeless. My husband kept saying we could stop, that it was ok if we didn't have children, that it could just be the two of us, but that was not at all what I wanted. I felt that to "complete" myself and my life, I needed to have children. I could feel that maternal clock ticking, and it was ticking hard!

We met with our Fertility Endocrinologist before our second procedure with the second set of eggs. My medicines were even amped up more this time. And, yet again, I had few eggs and only one was left after the 5-day waiting period. One egg was left, but it was a Level A. Hallelujah! I was pregnant! I couldn't believe it! Once again, I cried and cried, but this time "happy tears." I immediately called my husband and best friend. I didn't want to tell many people, because what if something happened? After all, could this really result in a real pregnancy? I was labeled high risk for a while. I was super cautious with everything I did. Nine months later, I had my beautiful baby girl. To this day, I would do it all over again.

* * *

147

There are also some seriously funny blogs on the real story of IVF, but the not-so-funny truth is that symptoms include exaggerated PMS, bruising from all the needles, sleepless nights, volatile mood from all the hormones, and a general weariness. Daily injections and hours spent at the doctor's office are the physical realities of IVF treatment cycles. The emotional realities are just as hard.

Natural Solutions for Fertility

I asked a natural family expert, Mandi Sanders, what she recommended to women who were struggling with fertility. She named "clean foods," meaning organic and unprocessed. She encourages women who are trying to conceive to include in their diets traditional foods, particularly pasture raised meats and organ meats that provide many of the vitamins and nutrients needed by women trying to become pregnant. She also recommended the following herbs: chaste tree, red clover blossoms, oat straw, nettles, and Shatavari. All of these have a long history of supporting the female reproductive system.

A reproductive endocrinologist friend of ours recommended the book *The Fertility Diet: Groundbreaking Research Reveals Natural Ways to Boost Ovulation and Improve Your Chances of Getting Pregnant*. This book explains, in laymen's terms, how food impacts hormone function.

The Riordan Clinic also has a You Tube video called *Natural Solutions to Infertility* on balancing the whole body system. It provides a good overview of practical, natural solutions. Additionally, *Taking Charge of Your Fertility* is the landmark work by Toni Weschler. Millions of women have prepared their bodies for pregnancy with the information in this paramount book. Based on these sources, if I were desperate to get pregnant, I would throw gluten out the window immediately.

Acupuncture and TCM (traditional Chinese medicine) have received the most attention of all the alternative therapies available for women struggling with fertility. One study showed that women undergoing acupuncture were more likely to become pregnant with IVF, according to C. Wanjek. Another study showed that acupuncture actually helps increase egg production as effectively as the fertility drug Clomid, according to C. Bouchez, writing on WebMD.

Consider these statistics from L. Carpenter's article in *The Guardian* about Dr. Xia-Ping Zhai in London who practices TCM: "Between 1995 and 2000 she had treated 224 patients (average age 37) with traditional Chinese medicine (TCM). After treatment for at least six months 76 percent of the women had become pregnant. Of these pregnancies, 77 percent resulted in a baby, and of the 23 percent who miscarried, 69 percent went on to have a baby later. In 2000 the fertility clinic at the very top of the Human Fertilisation and Embryology Authority league table was claiming a success rate of up to 38.8 percent. Zhai's success was in the 70s," according to L. Carpenter in *The Guardian.*

One of the main symptoms acupuncture manages is stress, which can greatly impact hormone levels throughout the body. Acupuncture and TCM are affordable solutions many women swear by. In the *Guardian*, Dr. Zhai says, "I've seen so many women. I know what I do works." While Western medicine cannot explain how acupuncture or TCM work, it would not hurt to keep an open mind.

Because fertility affects the emotions so strongly, there are dozens of "snake oil salesmen" on the internet who claim to have the solution or supplement that "cures" infertility. Be careful and do your own research. The consensus in alternative fertility solutions seems to focus on balancing the body's systems and hormones to support fertility. Information on balancing hormones and improving overall health consistently points to similar foods, supplements, and lifestyle changes that are manageable. If you seek an alternative healthcare practitioner, ask for reviews and do your own investigating. There are reputable alternatives available if you select them carefully.

Coping with Infertility

About half of all people who seek help for infertility never achieve fertility. For many women, an ongoing grieving process is attached to resigning themselves to life without children. The grief is as real as any death of a child. It is the death of a hoped-for child. A friend who was never able to conceive said the grief never ends. She is now in her mid-fifties and says there will be moments when she hears about a child graduating from college, and the pain is intense. When she hears of friends who have a first grandchild, the entire life of a never-born child flashes before her.

Our culture is conflicted. On one hand, we are among the least supportive cultures of motherhood; on the other, we expect women to be physical mothers. These expectations are hard on women who never have children. Childless women often report feeling less "womanly" and less "whole." There is no way to avoid the pain and grieving process. I want to share an excerpt from a blog written by L. O-Pries on coping with infertility: "This week and every week after, I want you to understand how infertility sucks people, couples, and families into a vortex of grief, disappointment, and isolation. There are some days when I feel like the grief is so intense that I am going to run out of breath because my sobbing is so violent and the pain cuts so deep. One time after a negative test, I cried for three straight days, and I was afraid I would never stop crying. When I see someone announce a pregnancy with a dreaded ultrasound picture on Facebook, it's like someone sucker-punched me and I am rolling on the ground writhing in pain. How unfair it feels that my friends and family are welcoming their second children in the same amount of time that we have struggled for our first."

Here are the top blogs I found on infertility: *The Truth About Trying: Redbook's Infertility Video Series, The Infertility Diaries, In*

These Small Moments, Single Infertile Female: Now What?, Hannah Wept Sarah Laughed, and *Coming2Terms.* Finding a community seems to be the key to overcoming the grief of infertility.

One of the most vibrant women I know has no children. I talked with her about this section, and she said, "You learn to thrive as *you.* Your life doesn't end. You cope. You use your other strengths and find joy in other places." She recommended a website called *Gateway Women.* The introduction reads:

> One in five women in the UK, Ireland, USA, Canada & Australia are now reaching their mid-forties without having had children, double what it was a generation ago. Although some women have actively chosen not to be mothers "childfree," many of us are "childless-by-circumstance" and find ourselves living a life we never planned for, and for which no one's got a roadmap!
>
> I set up Gateway Women in 2011 with the aim of supporting, inspiring, and empowering childless-by-circumstance women. To end our isolation and create a safe place for us to talk about our situation, work through our grief and sadness, and come out the other side ready to create a "Plan B" for a meaningful and fulfilling life without children. One that ROCKS!
>
> My book *Rocking the Life Unexpected: 12 Weeks to Your Plan B for a Meaningful and Fulfiling Life Without Children* was published in September 2013 and went to #1 on Amazon Kindle on day one!
>
> Please do join our private online community. It's only been going since December 2012, and it's already been reviewed as the best in the world. It's inclusive, non-judgmental, wise, friendly, and funny. "Support for the hard stuff; enthusiasm for the good stuff" is how one member described it.
>
> It's not just you this has happened to. There's nothing wrong with you, and you didn't screw up. Welcome to Gateway Women. Welcome, finally, to YOUR tribe.

Women sharing their stories and becoming Mothers in a metaphorical sense is powerful. These women become Mothers to projects, adventures, causes, and other people. They carry the same archetype characteristics as physical mothers into the world, and we need more of them to share their gifts within communities.

If you are a woman still coping with the grief of a child that was never born, I urge you to find a community that values The Mother in all women, and know you are not alone. Giving physical birth to a child is not a precursor to Motherhood, and as I have written from the beginning of this book, the world needs more Mothers. Let us share your pain and grief, but let us also help you transform it into what our world really needs, which is courageous, strong, caring Mothers.

What is Causing Infertility To Impact So Many Women?

While the rising age in women trying to conceive is among the most common candidates for infertility, it is not the only one. Environmental factors that have been associated with decreased fertility include cigarette smoke, radiation, dry cleaning chemicals, and lead. Pesticides are also receiving frequent coverage lately as culprits for decreased fertility.

Women who live near crops on which particular pesticides have been used may have anywhere from a 40 to 120 percent increased risk of miscarriage, according to Fertility Factor.

While I do not feel qualified to speak to the damages these factors cause, or the significance of their impact, I would like to acknowledge that the chemicals we are exposed to on a daily basis could have a significant impact on our health. The best book I can recommend on the subject is *The Autoimmune Epidemic* by Donna Jackson Nakagawa which is an intensely investigative documentation of how environmental factors impact our immune systems overall.

I also suggest the website and app *Skin Deep*. It is an informative site, provided by the *Environmental Working Group*, that details analysis of the chemicals and toxins contained in common personal care products that can impact your fertility and your health. Find out just how harmful your shampoo may really be by scanning the barcode at the store with your phone. *The Collaborative on Health and the Environment* website provides a clear body of research on how environmental factors impact infertility and related reproductive disorder.

Many integrative physicians believe that the rise in infertility is most likely caused by hormone imbalances resulting from lifestyle and environmental factors. Many women are in a constant state of estrogen dominance. According to Justin Marchegiani of *Primal Docs*, women who struggle with fertility should look into hormonal imbalances as a real source of the problem. He recommends stabilizing hormones and blood sugar, avoiding common toxins and chemicals in make-up, hygiene, and cleaning products. Getting your hormone levels checked is a good place to start.

Again, I bring up this topic because I do not think it gets enough attention. Numerous field studies link environmental contaminants to a whole range of reproductive abnormalities in wildlife and to reduced reproductive rates and population size. These data come from many species, including birds, fish, mollusks and mammals. These studies demonstrate quite clearly the impact environmental exposure to chemicals has caused on animals, according to Resolve: The National Infertility Association.

Why are we so careless with what we expose ourselves to as humans? Why aren't more studies being done on the long-term impact of chemicals we have become dependent on like glyphosate in Round-up? Why does it feel taboo to ask these questions in the doctor's office even if our very basic ability to create life depends on them? These are questions I believe we need to bring to the table now so that future generations are not left wondering what we were thinking.

Our cultural expectations for women regarding Motherhood significantly impact our feelings about fertility and infertility. Struggling to have a child and struggling with the realities of not having a child are core issues for women in the Mother archetype phase. Because fertility is so central to women's identities, we need to keep asking critical questions about what factors help or hurt our ability to carry a healthy child to term.

We also need to keep expanding roles of women who do not have children. Motherhood does not have to mean giving physical birth to a physical child. How many of us are indebted to women other than our physical mothers for helping shape our lives, our communities, and our worlds in important ways? Nel Noddings calls this "The Ethic of Care," which she says, when it dominates, turns our world into a very different place than our competitive, every-man-for-himself, "Ethic of Justice." The Mother archetype calls each one of us to create, to cultivate, and to care.

Chapter 9
Pregnancy & Birth Options

"Many women have described their experiences of childbirth as being associated with a spiritual uplifting, the power of which they have never previously been aware. To such a woman, childbirth is a monument of joy within her memory. She turns to it in thought to seek again an ecstasy which passed too soon."
—Grantly Dick Read

"Later on Lady Maccon was to describe that particular day as the worst of her life. She had neither the soul nor the romanticism to consider childbirth magical or emotionally transporting. So far as she could gather it mostly involved pain, indignity, and mess. There was nothing engaging or appealing about the process. And as she told her husband firmly she intended never to go through it again."
–Gail Carriger

There are so many things I wish I knew during the pregnancies of my babies and their births that I know now. I did pretty well. I bought every pregnancy book I could find. I took prenatal vitamins; although, I did not start them until I got pregnant. I did not drink, except for a glass of wine on my third pregnancy at a holiday party.

I avoided tuna and other mercury-containing fish and never ate sushi. I exercised right up until my due date, at least during the first pregnancy. My husband even changed the cat litter throughout my pregnancies, even though he hated the cat.

Being pregnant was the healthiest I had ever been. But there are some things I wish I had known that go beyond the typical OB/GYN advice and the standard advice in *What to Expect....* I want to talk

155

about these harder to find things in this chapter.

There is no way I would tell another woman how to have a baby. When Mike and I became pregnant with our first child, I got that Christmas Eve feeling every time I thought about it, but adjusting to the reality of a baby coming took some doing.

We had our share of moodiness, misunderstandings, and all-out fights during our journey, but when it came down to it, giving birth to Max was the second best day of my life.

I really didn't have strong feelings either way about how I would deliver my child. I figured I would get an epidural and glide through the whole experience as painlessly as possible. I signed Mike and myself up for a birthing class at the hospital where he was a resident. Our teacher gave one of the most balanced classes anywhere. Although I didn't know it at the time, she, herself, had delivered her babies at a birthing center across the street, but had no problem talking about the advantages of hospital births. I remember her describing all the possible pain control methods, and while she must have had strong feelings against them, given her own choices, I never knew it. She did recommend a birthing ball, a giant green exercise ball that Mike was teased by his fellow residents for carrying around the hospital while I was in labor.

You sit on a birthing ball during pregnancy and labor and roll it under your hips to help them open. She also encouraged us to bring music into the birthing room and gave us a thing that smelled good when it heated up on a light bulb in the room. I had no idea these things weren't perfectly standard practice in hospital births!

Our birth teacher guided us through writing a birthing plan. We sat down with the seriousness of writing a will and wrote out what we wanted to happen during our birthing process. After much consideration, Mike and I decided on a natural birth as long as possible, and then possibly, an epidural. I wanted to nurse my child immediately, and I didn't want the baby to leave the room.

Mike was scheduled to take his board exams in another state two days after my due date. I panicked at the thought of giving birth without him there, so the day before I was due, I asked about induction. I told the doctor my reason, and he wrote the order. I came in the next night at 5 p.m. to begin Pitocin.

I did not do any research on induced labor. I didn't even see any conflict with my natural birth plan and speeding up the process a bit. My mom came in just as my contractions started coming really hard the next morning.

At ten that morning, I had not dilated at all, so the doctor broke my water. Max had meconium, which meant he had passed a bowel movement in the womb. I learned about the concern for inhaling meconium and started to get a little nervous. As much as I walked and rolled on my birthing ball, I did not dilate.

My contractions were horrid. At noon I decided I needed that epidural after all. The resident missed with that huge needle. An hour later I was writhing in pain with no relief and no dilation. The nurse said, "The epidural must not have taken," and she ran to find an attending doctor. In the meantime, they gave me some pain medicine through the IV that made me loopy. "Crocodile Rock" blared on my birthing playlist.

I yelled at Mike, "Who put this annoying song on here!"

Finally, the attending doctor came, and the second epidural provided much needed relief. I calmed down and focused my energy on my stubborn cervix. At four in the afternoon, I was still not dilating, and I could tell my husband was getting nervous.

Max was showing signs of distress on all the fetal monitors. The doctor said it was time to consider a c-section. That was not in the birthing plan. I wanted to wait a little longer. The doctor said, "Would you rather risk a serious complication, or get that baby out here safely?"

At 4:30 they wheeled me into the OR and the anesthesiologist started "saddle block" anesthesia to numb me from the chest down.

At 5:30 p.m., I got to kiss Max on his sweet little forehead since my neck was the only part of my body that I could move. By six, I was nursing and falling deeply in love. I had never in my life been more exhausted.

Nutrition During Pregnancy

According to the Mayo Clinic, food impacts pregnancy more than you might realize. They include on their list of foods to avoid: seafood high in mercury (1/2 of a can of tuna per week is considered too much), raw or undercooked seafood or meat, unpasteurized foods, caffeine, some herbal teas, alcohol, and unwashed fruits and vegetables.

Mayo recommends prenatal vitamins containing the following ingredients: Folic acid — 400 to 800 micrograms, Calcium — 250 milligrams, Iron — 30 milligrams, Vitamin C — 50 milligrams, Zinc — 15 milligrams, Copper — 2 milligrams, Vitamin B-6 — 2 milligrams, Vitamin D — 400 international units.

Several supplements, which I learned about after having babies, are missing from this list, such as Omega 3s which are brain food. Low levels of Omega 3 fats have been implicated in every disorder from ADHD to heart disease to depression.

Omega 3s optimize brain growth in children, especially during the third trimester. However, since most Omega 3s come from fish oil, and most fish is high in mercury, the best place to get these important building blocks during pregnancy is Krill oil. Krill are tiny sea animals that contain antioxidants and less mercury. Another good source is grass-fed beef.

When cattle eat grass, they produce Omega 3s that are absent in the meat of grain-fed cows, according to J.M. Mercola. Vitamin D is another important supplement. In pregnant and postpartum women, vitamin D deficiency has been associated with depression and poor obstetrical outcomes including low birth weight, maternal preeclampsia, hypertension, and gestational diabetes, according to

Kelly Brogan.

Women who take high doses of vitamin D during pregnancy have a greatly reduced risk of complications, including gestational diabetes, preterm birth, and infection.

In order to reach these benefits, it is recommended that pregnant women take 4,000 international units of vitamin D every day, which is 10 times the amount available in most prenatal vitamins. Women in one study at the Medical University of South Carolina who took 4,000 IU of the vitamin daily in their second and third trimesters showed no evidence of harm, but they had half the rate of pregnancy-related complications as women who took 400 IU of vitamin D every day, according to S. Boyles on webmd.com.

Probiotics during pregnancy are recommended by everyone from Dr. Sears to Dr. Mercola to WebMD. The most recent understanding of how a healthy dose of good guys in the digestive tract impacts a myriad of health concerns is astounding. In a recent article from the *Huffington Post*, the author claims that the use of probiotics during pregnancy impacts digestive health, urinary health, allergies, reproductive health, immunity, and even obesity. They may even have a role in decreasing skin allergies.

These are among the pieces of information I wish I had known. I was a vegetarian during my first two pregnancies, something I now consider pretty unhealthy the way I practiced it. And while I took prenatal vitamins, I wish I had ingested tons of probiotics and enough vitamin D. These are the things I will know when my daughter starts a family.

Environmental Concerns

It is easy to write off environmental concerns because they are usually invisible, and we live under a false sense of belief that our government agencies are regulating harmful agents.

Consider this excerpt from an article in *Scientific American* by P. Hunt: "Susan starts her day by jogging to the edge of town, cutting back through a cornfield for an herbal tea at the downtown Starbucks and heading home for a shower. It sounds like a healthy morning routine, but Susan is in fact exposing herself to a rogue's gallery of chemicals: pesticides and herbicides on the corn, plasticizers in her tea cup, and the wide array of ingredients used to perfume her soap and enhance the performance of her shampoo and moisturizer. Most of these exposures are so low as to be considered trivial, but they are not trivial at all—especially considering that Susan is six weeks pregnant."

The author states that an increasing number of clinicians and scientists are becoming convinced that these chemical exposures contribute to obesity, endometriosis, diabetes, autism, allergies, cancer, and other diseases. Dozens of agencies and experts have called for legislation to require chemical companies to prove their products are safe before marketing them, but as of yet, there is no protocol for doing this.

By now, everybody knows smoking cigarettes and using illicit drugs during pregnancy is awful for fetal development, but there are a host of other substances that can have significant impacts on your baby's fetal health. They don't have a bad smell or visible fumes attached to them, and it is hard to keep up with the latest research on the worst offenders. In fact, I am almost glad I didn't know about things like endocrine disruptors when I was pregnant. They are everywhere, and I might never have slept!

The Department of Women's Health encourages pregnant women to avoid exposure to lead, mercury, arsenic, pesticides, solvents, and cigarette smoke. These are the typical warnings every doctor and pregnancy book will give you. However, the even more sinister candidates are endocrine disruptors. They are in everything from pesticides and household cleaners to plastics and carpets. They mimic hormones and wreak havoc on young fetus development that cannot be seen until years later.

Some of the country's leading toxicologists recently published their findings on endocrine disruptors and strongly urge our government to take action on regulating their use. I read a powerful piece in the *New York Times* by N. Kristof about how knowledge of endocrine disruptors changed behaviors in a leading researcher. To protect his own family, he stopped buying canned food, stopped microwaving in plastic containers, and quit using pesticides because of his research on this subject.

Trying to avoid all the potential pitfalls of environmental dangers for our unborn can be overwhelming, but if the leading researcher on endocrine disruptors is disturbed, shouldn't we pay attention, too? The good news is that there are things you can do to mitigate the effects of bad stuff in our environment.

Beauty Products: There is a great app for your phone called *Skin Deep*. You can scan the bar code of most cosmetics and personal beauty products to find out their safety rating by the Environmental Working Group. I use it every time I buy toothpaste, shampoo, soap, make-up or sunscreen. Pick the products with ratings of 0-2, and find alternatives to the rest. Dr. Bronner's Soap is what I use head to toe in the shower and on the kids.

Household Cleaners: Vinegar cleans nearly everything, and it is cheap. There are dozens of recipes for homemade cleaning supplies online for everything from wood floors to bathrooms. Find the one or two that work for you, and use them on everything. If you have money to spare, check out the Environmental Working Group's website for information on the safest commercial cleaners available on the market.

Remodeling: Low VOC paint is available most everywhere now, but it wouldn't hurt to let your girlfriends or family paint the nursery as a gift for the new baby. Many expectant parents think they need to remodel, but tearing up floors or scraping wallpaper exposes you to all kinds of airborne toxins that your baby doesn't need. If you have to clean something, wear a mask.

Food: There is really no reason every family cannot eat healthy, organic food in this country. I have heard millions of excuses, but I do not buy them. Find a local farmer, go to your farmer's market, or buy things when they are in season and cheap and then freeze them. I have a friend whose family does a Work Share for a box of fresh organic veggies from a local farmer. They give time to the farm and get veggies in return.

If you are pressed for time, look on the Environmental Working Group's Dirty Dozen list and find out which vegetables and fruits are the most essential to buy organic, and which ones might be okay to buy treated. Almost all farmer's markets now accept SNAP benefits and EBT cards.

Grow your own. You can rent a plot in a community garden if you don't have a yard. Communities are practically giving these away due to lack of use! Take a gardening class. Read a book. Ask old-timers who still know how to produce their own food. Get on the internet and look it up. Producing your own food provides financial and health benefits that are astounding.

Stay away from any plastic container that is not labeled "BPA-free" explicitly. Skip canned goods; the inside lining is bad news for chemicals. If you do use plastics, look for the ones with recycle numbers 4 and 5 on the bottom. Please don't microwave plastic. And store food in glass containers or jars.

Cell Phones: More and more research is coming out on cell phones. The concerns span from behavioral problems to wireless radiation exposure, but I do not know enough to comment on the subject. I know if I were to get pregnant now, I would look into it. The shift in usage is significant since I have had my children. We don't even have a home phone now. I would want to know the latest research.

Antioxidants: There are numerous studies on how antioxidants mitigate the effects of harmful toxins in the body. Micronutrients from vitamins and food can be beneficial to developing babies by fighting off carcinogens and endocrine disruptors. Increasing the number of foods you consume that are high in antioxidants can help counter some of the exposure we have to an onslaught of harmful chemicals. Dr. Oz's recommendations for eating a rainbow of food are helpful. He recommends green foods for vitamin C, E quercetin (a flavonoid), and sulforaphane.

Dr. Wahls (from the Preface) extols including seaweed in your diet to rid the body of toxins. Just one cup, or a fist-size portion, of green foods per day provides plenty of antioxidants. Cruciferous veggies such as broccoli, spinach, escarole, and parsley contain isothiocyanates (ITCs), which are important for detoxification. Fruits and veggies that are bright yellow and orange contain vitamin A, which helps maintain healthy organs and prevents bacteria from growing. Vitamin A also helps prevent cancer, heart disease, high blood pressure, and even depression, according to K. Kirkpatrick on doctoroz.com.

How you cook matters. According to the Rodale Institute, over-cooking kills nutrients in green foods, such as broccoli. Never microwave broccoli because the intense heat drains all of the nutrients. The same goes for boiling; you'll notice the water turns green. The color is where all the nutrients are. Chop florets in half or quarters to get the healthful enzymes to emerge. Cook carrots whole; cutting them allows more nutrients to escape.

When cooking sweet potatoes, bake, broil, or steam. The nutrients are contained when the potato is cooked in its own skin. Wild salmon is great for added antioxidants. Baking, broiling, poaching, and steaming are the best methods to cook salmon. Frying salmon or any fish will sap the nutrients. Grilling salmon on an outdoor grill can add cancer-causing heterocyclic amines, or HCAs. If you crave grilled salmon, adding rosemary before grilling may actually combat HCA production.

What you eat, where it comes from, and how it is prepared determine your food quality. High food quality is one of the most important and overlooked factors in creating optimum health.

Behavior During Pregnancy

Your behaviors do change a lot during pregnancy on their own, but some things are a bit counterintuitive. Sleep becomes critical for moms and developing babies but is sometimes harder to get. Exercise is important but can be uncomfortable. Women on antidepressants and other medications may have legitimate concerns about how their medications will affect their baby's health.

Sleep: During each of my three pregnancies, I could have slept ten hours a night and then taken a nap, no problem. This didn't mean I stayed asleep all night, just that I was always tired. I remember looking for some sleep aid that was okay to take during pregnancy because I knew if I woke up during the night, I might not make it through the next day.

When I was pregnant, doctors recommended Tylenol PM or Benadryl for sleep, and I believe they still do. Other recommendations include concluding exercise at least four hours before bedtime and eating high carbohydrate foods and high protein foods for good dreams. Emptying your bladder before bedtime is also a frequent recommendation, along with sleeping with extra pillows between your legs or supporting your back.

However, before you rush to the drugstore to buy an over-the-counter sleep medication, consider one of the following natural sleep remedies, recommended by mercola.com. They are safer and have fewer side effects. Many of these cannot only help you fall asleep and stay asleep, but they can also promote muscle relaxation. Magnesium and calcium are both sleep aids, and when taken together, they become even more effective. By taking magnesium, you cancel out any potential heart problems that might arise from taking calcium alone.

Take 200 milligrams of magnesium (you can lower the dose if it causes diarrhea) and 600 milligrams of calcium each night. Aromatherapy is another option. Lavender is the most well-known. It is non-toxic and soothing. Find a spray with real lavender and spritz it onto your pillow before bedtime, or buy a lavender-filled pillow. Choose gentle yoga or stretching for exercise to help sleep. Try easy yoga stretches in bed followed by simple meditation. Close your eyes and, for 5 to 10 minutes, pay attention to nothing but your breathing.

Exercise: Physical fitness is very important during pregnancy, even though you may not feel like moving. In fact, it may be the last thing you feel like doing, so do not push yourself too hard. Just make movement a priority. Park farther away from the grocery store or work than you normally would. Buy a pregnancy yoga tape. Take a prenatal exercise class if you can find one.

Stretch, get outside, and walk. I had a huge belly from the start of my pregnancies. It stuck straight out, and exercise hurt! I found something called a pregnancy belt that wrapped around my lower back and belly and fastened under my huge bump. I wore that thing through three pregnancies when I worked out or traveled, and it was worth every penny. If you do feel strong, there is no reason to slow your routine. Just listen to your body.

Medication: When it comes to medications during pregnancy, most women have to weigh the consequences. Many women make the decision that a depressed mom is worse for their children than the possible side effects of anti-depressants. There are many different medications that could negatively impact a developing fetus and many more that just haven't been significantly tested. The best rule of thumb with pregnancy is the more natural, the better. We simply do not fully understand all the ways chemicals, environmental factors, and medications impact growth and development, and as any mom will tell you, you do not want to look back and regret a short-term decision.

Nutrition: Many pregnancy illnesses and ailments can be prevented with nutrition. I was still treating symptoms when I was pregnant with my three kids. I hope to impart to you how to take care of your body so that many of the symptoms will not occur to begin with. I want to end this section with advice from herbalist Susun Weed, who writes in susunweed.com: "Wise women believe that most of the problems of pregnancy can be prevented by attention to nutrition. Morning sickness and mood swings are connected to low blood sugar; backaches and severe labor pains often result from insufficient calcium; varicose veins, hemorrhoids, constipation, skin discoloration and anemia are evidence of lack of specific nutrients; preeclampsia, the most severe problem of pregnancy, is a form of acute malnutrition. Excellent nutrition includes pure water, controlled breath, abundant light, loving and respectful relationships, beauty and harmony in daily life, joyous thoughts and vital foodstuffs."

Weed recommends red raspberry leaves brewed as an infusion as the safest of all uterine and pregnancy tonic herbs. Red raspberry leaves contain fragarine, which helps tone muscles, and a rich concentration of vitamins A, B, C, and E, and provides easily assimilated iron and calcium. Red raspberry leaf in combination with red clover increases fertility in men and women. She also recommends nettle leaves, which contain almost every vitamin and mineral necessary for human health and growth.

Supporting overall health with supplies of vitamins and minerals through quality sources of food or supplements is a cornerstone of fertility and pregnancy. Avoiding and mitigating the effects of harmful environmental elements is another important factor. We cannot expect our reproductive systems to go unchanged by such an upsurge in chemicals. It is our responsibility as a culture to deal honestly and skeptically with the cost-benefit of our easy lifestyle afforded by the chemicals we use every day and have come to depend on.

Birthing Options
From home births to planned cesareans, women's choices about

how to give birth in the United States have never been greater. While there are tensions around issues of birthing legalities, such as the ability to practice midwifery or operate birthing centers, information on safely birthing children in a variety of situations is growing. Between 1990 and 2004, according to the CDC, the percentage of U.S. births that occurred at home increased by 29 percent. However, the vast majority of births in the U.S. still occur in hospitals.

What I want to advocate for in this writing is doing our own research and asking tough questions. For example, why is the rate of cesarean births so much higher in the United States than in other developed countries? What are the success and complication rates of trained midwives? What long-term effects on our children do our birthing choices create? Which medical interventions are necessary? What improvements do we need to make in birthing practices? How does our culture shape our decisions?

I believe we are moving in the right direction. We are bringing critically high standards to natural birth practitioners. We are also beginning to reclaim the natural process of birth in hospitals. In our own local hospital, the OB/GYNs are now familiar with doulas (birthing coaches or assistants), keeping babies in the room with the mother following birth, and post-birth practices that promote breastfeeding. The pendulum is beginning to swing toward a healthy middle that includes scientifically trained midwives and compassionately trained physicians.

Medical Interventions at Birth

Medical interventions during birth have saved countless lives. They have made birthing a joyful endeavor more often than the terrifying brush with death it used to be for most women. However, in recent years, a backlash toward medical births has grown, and for good reason.

The World Health Organization recommends optimal rates of c-sections at 5 to 10 percent of the population. In 2010, cesarean rates in the US leveled off at 32.8 percent, according to childbirthconnection.org. Women have begun to feel like medicine has robbed them of their natural ability to birth. Families have started to question medical advice and practices received in hospitals critically, rather than accepting recommendations blindly. Women are beginning to understand that painless births come with hidden trade-offs.

Pitocin: Taking Pitocin to speed up my labor probably ensured a c-section for me. I might have ended up with one anyway, but women who take Pitocin are more than twice as likely to have a c-section. It also produces harder labor, which increases the likelihood of the need for pain management. The U.S. Pitocin package insert lists these warnings:

- fetal heart abnormalities (slow heartbeat, PVCs and arrhythmias)
- low APGAR scores
- neonatal jaundice
- neonatal retinal hemorrhage
- permanent central nervous system or brain damage
- fetal death

That is a long list of increased risks. I was aware of exactly zero of them when I elected to receive Pitocin in order to avoid delivering my first child while my husband was away. I take full responsibility for not doing my own homework. I wanted to have the baby when I wanted to have him. I never weighed the risks.

Epidural: Epidurals are routinely used during labor. They have been termed a laboring woman's best friend. I know lots of women who swore by their epidurals and many who mourned the fact that they waited too long to receive one. Epidurals can make labor more comfortable while keeping women lucid throughout the process. There are, however, possible side effects. Epidurals have been shown to have the following effects on labor and laboring mothers, according to Chris Kresser.

They lengthen labor, triple the risk of severe perineal tear, increase risk of cesarean section by 2.5 times, and triple the occurrence of induction with oxytocin. Epidurals quadruple the chances a baby will be face-up in the final stages of labor and decrease the chance of spontaneous vaginal delivery by almost half. In addition, epidurals increase the chances of complications from instrument delivery and increase risk of pelvic floor problems following delivery.

C-sections: We live in a culture where elective surgeries are normal. C-sections don't seem like such a big deal in this context. Undoubtedly, they have saved countless lives and are sometimes medical necessities. What I want to convey here is that, even when they may be the best option, c-sections shouldn't be undertaken lightly. The complications associated with cesarean sections for even low-risk, healthy babies are numerous.

Complications include increased risk of respiratory compromise, low blood sugar, and poor temperature regulation. Babies who are born through cesarean demonstrate slower neurological adaptations after birth, increased risk of oxidative stress, and depressed immune function.

There are differences in levels of hormones regulating calcium metabolism, renin-angiotensin, progesterone, creatine kinase, dopamine, nitric oxide synthesis, thyroid hormones and liver enzymes. The most significant and lasting risk for babies delivered via cesarean is the alteration of gut flora.

Studies have consistently shown that cesarean babies have altered fecal microbial make-ups compared with vaginally born babies, which can persist for six months and quite possibly for life. One of my favorite, well- researched series on childbirth is by Chris Kresser. Here is an excerpt from an article on cesarean sections:

Rethinking Women's Health

Among other things, the gut flora promotes normal gastrointestinal function, provides protection from infection, regulates metabolism and comprises more than 75 percent of our immune system.

Dysregulated gut flora has been linked to diseases ranging from autism and depression to autoimmune conditions like Hashimoto's, inflammatory bowel disease and type 1 diabetes. This probably explains why babies born via cesarean may have increased susceptibility to gut infections, asthma and allergies later in life.

The marked changes in gut flora in cesarean babies are not greatly affected by the method of feeding (i.e. breastfeeding vs. formula) afterwards. This means that breastfeeding after cesarean section can't compensate for the alterations in gut flora experienced with that type of delivery.

If you did have a cesarean for any reason, I recommend using a high-quality infant probiotic to help populate your baby's gut with beneficial flora. The brand I use in my practice is called Therbiotic Infant, from Klaire labs. (Important note: although they recommend starting with 1/4 tsp, that is far too high of a dose. I suggest lightly dusting the nipple with the powder once or twice a day before feedings. If you notice diarrhea, especially with green flecks or tint, decrease the dose.)

As I said earlier, I am thankful I have three healthy children. I am thankful to the doctors who delivered them as safely as they knew how. I am thankful I was unscathed, for the most part, by my pregnancies. What I regret is that I did not know any of the information listed above. We do not get to make these decisions over again, and knowing the real costs and benefits of our decisions is important.

170

V-bacs (vaginal birth after cesarean)

I was told, by my OB/GYN, that giving birth within two years of a c-section meant that you needed to have another section because the uterus had not had time to fully heal and might rupture. We became pregnant with Ben 10 months after Max was born, and I didn't question her advice. And then, when we had Cecelia, I had another section because I had heard, "If you've had two, you better just have another."

I am sure the advice was sound in my case, but it wasn't the only advice I could have received. V-bacs are possible, but I did not have the information on the good bacteria my babies were missing out on by skipping the birth canal to motivate me to try to find out about them. Max had been healthy, and, while I felt a little robbed of my birth experience, I preferred a healthy delivery.

It was not until my kids started getting ear infections every other month, despite the fact that I nursed them all for a year, that I started to question why their immune systems were so weak. It wasn't until I read an article, when my third child was a year old, on the important chemicals that the mom releases to the baby just before the baby enters the world that I started to second-guess my decision. I wish I had at least tried a v-bac. It might not have worked, but in the scenario of a hospital birth, I think the risk might have been worth it.

Vaginal births after a cesarean are rare, due in part to cultural misunderstandings. The result is a 90 percent repeat cesarean rate in America. The big risk of a ruptured uterus that women worry about is, in reality, about 0.5-1 percent according to J. Kamel's article "Myths About VBAC." A more accurate understanding of v-bacs might be that all births are susceptible to complications, but doctors and hospitals have protocols to deal with each one. There are doctors who are more comfortable with v-bacs than others. Find one who will talk with you objectively about your options.

Natural Birth

Natural birth is on the rise, and for good reason. Lots of women are beginning to question the extent of intervention in traditional hospitals. They want to reclaim the very natural ability to have a child. Most of my friends from other countries did not use epidurals, although they had their babies in a hospital setting. Also, a growing number of women I meet have had home births, used midwives or doulas, and claim birthing as the most powerful experience on earth.

They trust their body's ability to do its job with the guidance of other experienced women and family members. They want birth to be experienced fully, because it is simply more powerful that way, and, many believe, healthier for the baby.

These women write books, publish magazines, teach classes, and provide online support in the face of an industrialized healthcare system that does not generally promote their efforts. The legal issues alone for using midwives and birthing centers are daunting. The liability for midwives would frighten the most lion-hearted, yet they persist, and they appear to be growing stronger.

I applaud the work that these women are doing to reclaim a natural, human, and conservative/judicial use of intervention in a birthing experience. Because of their efforts, things like kangaroo care (holding a premature newborn skin on skin to her mother's chest to increase heart rate) are infiltrating the medical model. Mothers keep their babies in their rooms now, instead of having them whisked away to a nursery. Breastfeeding is encouraged in almost every hospital. And physicians are becoming used to birthing plans, doulas, and even midwives.

Mandi Sanders, a natural family living teacher, shared her home birth story with me. She writes:

We welcomed our first baby into our hearts on Sunday July 8, at 9:29 p.m. I had some early signs of his arrival the Thursday night before as I was folding laundry and listening to music and

felt some contractions that were different from all the Braxton-Hicks ones I had been feeling. So, I did some yoga and belly dancing (well, kind of) to stretch through it. Of course I wasn't thinking that these were real contractions. They continued Friday and Saturday off and on. Will decided not to go to work Saturday night, just in case, and he cooked a wonderful dinner with a salad fresh from the garden and pasta full of yummies from the garden as well. We enjoyed spending what we knew were likely our last moments as just the two of us.

I woke up Sunday morning around 8 am hungry, of course. He made me some scrambled eggs and toast, my usual. Then, I went back to sleep and didn't wake until 11 am. That was the
latest I had slept in ages! Little did I realize that I needed to, for all the work that was in store for me later in the day.

I woke up because I had an awfully upset stomach. I went to the bathroom and realized that I was having some contractions as well. So, I asked Will to time them as I sat on the toilet. They were pretty regular for an hour or two, but I was stuck on the toilet. I decided around 1 pm to call the midwives as they had a good 90 minute drive. My midwife pretty much confirmed my thoughts that I was indeed in labor, but we all figured I had a ways to go with this being my first. We called my mom, and she, my dad, and my sis all headed over. I decided to put on some clothes and put on this awesome green earthy printed wrap cloth that I have had forever and really wanted to wear during labor.

And then, back to the toilet where I pretty much worked through every contraction. I was getting up to walk around and chit chat in between. Early labor was actually no big deal for me—just having a contraction and sitting on the toilet. It was so comfy for some reason!

Everyone had arrived by 4 pm, and after the midwives had settled in, one asked if she could check my progress. I was about 4 cm and 90 percent effaced. They (my midwife, her assistant, and their apprentice) decided to go into town and eat some dinner in order to give Will and me some time together.

They had been gone about 20 minutes when my water broke at 6:45pm. First, a lovely trickle down my leg in the hallway on my way to sit on the [sic] porcelain throne. My sweet black lab so kindly cleaned me off. Then, during the next contraction I thought I would try to find a new spot to labor and with a gush, the rest of the fluid rushed onto the bed. Luckily, my midwife had already covered it with one of the sets of sheets and plastic drop cloths. My mom called the midwife to let her know that they should probably turn around. Next thing I know I am completely in active labor—full force.

Melissa, my midwife's assistant suggests that I sit in the shower on the birthing ball because my throne was losing its appeal. As I stepped in, I felt the urge to push, and you could hear it in my voice. I heard my midwife, Kim, say, "Okay. Let's get you to where you want to be—it's time to have a baby!"

The next hour or so is blurry as everything was so intense and unknown to me, all happening so quickly. I recall puking on Corinne, my midwife's apprentice, as I stepped out of the shower and began walking to my bed. Melissa and Will supported me as I needed to squat through contractions at that point. She kept whispering kind and encouraging words in my ear. I recall them checking me to see that my cervix was not quite there. I had about a half a centimeter to go. However, my body was eagerly
pushing.

I tried many different positions to get comfortable. I ended up in a sideways position on the bed pushing with Will behind me as my chair, holding his and Kim's hands. After several good pushes, I felt the ring o' fire, and Kim was telling me to touch his
head. For some reason, I could not at first. I just could not reach down there.

And then I did.

It totally re-energized me to push his head on out. Next, the body was getting ready to come out. He did not restitute, and I was pushing him out football shoulders style. Luckily, there was no tearing at all (thanks to my midwives supporting my perineum with warm washcloths). It was the absolute best feeling in the world to push him out. The relief was immediate.

It was no orgasmic labor, but the actual birth definitely was! My mom caught him as Melissa unwrapped the umbilical cord from around his neck. Will looked at me through the tears in his eyes and whispered, "It's a boy!!"

All I could come up with was, "I was right!"

174

He was perfect!

Tripp cried and then he cried some more, and finally after 30 minutes of crying, he decided to latch on, and our babymoon began...

In less than three hours, I went from active labor, to transition, to pushing, to heaven. I couldn't believe it happened so fast. We all celebrated with some homemade strawberry cake my dad had been working on, along with a roasted herb chicken, brown rice and veggies. I was starving! My belly was even growling during the last couple of pushes, and I told myself not to get distracted by it.

Afterwards, Will and I lay there in our bed just looking at this beautiful little human we created. We were in awe for quite some time until we finally wound down and slept.

* * *

I asked a natural birthing coach to recommend resources for women interested in learning more about natural birth. She recommended *Mothering Magazine*, *Ina May's Guide to Childbirth*, and *Your Best Birth: Know All Your Options, Discover the Natural Choices*, and *Take Back the Birthing Experience*. She also recommended *Pushed: The Painful Truth about Childbirth and Modern Maternity Care*, and *Childbirth Without Fear*.

The Fourth Trimester

The fourth trimester is something I did not hear about until my second child had colic. The fourth trimester is the three-to-four-month transition period from the womb to the world. It is the period when mothers think that the joy and relief of giving birth is coming, and realize that the reality of hard work has just begun. According to Dr. Sears, babies who do not make this transition easily are labeled difficult. These babies need to be held more, nursed more, and they cry more.

This time is also difficult for many mothers. Lack of sleep, hormonal changes, and identity shifts are all a part of new motherhood that is shocking for some new mothers. According to the Mayo Clinic, post-baby powerful emotions can range from joy, to "baby blues," to longer-lasting depression.

Typical symptoms include mood swings, anxiety, sadness, irritability, feeling overwhelmed, and crying. Indications of more severe post-partum depression include difficulty bonding with the baby, anxiety attacks, excessive crying, and withdrawing from friends and family. Post partum depression is caused by the biochemical and hormonal changes that happen in the body after pregnancy and birth. Antidepressants are normally prescribed if mood does not improve within a week or two.

The fourth trimester is particularly hard for young mothers because of our current family structure and social and professional support. Many women are isolated in their care for a new baby. Surrounding yourself with family and friends is important. Take breaks, get out of the house, join a new mom's group like La Leche League, invite people from your place of worship to help, and take care of yourself. Eating well, getting rest, and asking for help are keys to surviving the fourth trimester. Most importantly, new mothers need to know this three-four month adjustment period is normal.

We are living in the most incredible time to give birth. We have more live, safe births than ever before in the history of humans. We are afforded the ability of looking critically at our practices and asking what is best for our babies, long-term. We possess the knowledge and courage to make birthing practices even better as long as we do our homework and advocate for our babies, rather than following cultural trends in birthing impulsively. How we bring our babies into the world is an important step in beginning their care.

Chapter 10
Caregiving & Motherhood

"I imagine a new America in which citizens recognize that providers of physical, intellectual, emotional, and spiritual care are as indispensable to our society and our economy as providers of income."
—Anne Marie Slaughter

I think there are probably a dozen arrangements for raising children that benefit their emotional, spiritual, intellectual, and physical growth. I also know caregiving is not valued in our competitive culture. In every profession, the people who do the most direct, hands-on care are the lowest on the totem pole.

For example: college professors and preschool teachers, physicians and nurse's assistants, chefs and cafeteria workers, engineers and housecleaners. The people in our society who are most directly tied to physical care jobs (cleaning, fixing, cooking, changing diapers, wiping noses, bathing patients) have the least desirable and least well-compensated jobs.

Whether it is stay-at-home moms or dads, daycare workers, grandparents, or institutions, caring for children is not a highly recognized or rewarded position, yet it is so vitally important! It took me a long time to value mothering. I valued teaching. I valued education. But I did not value myself as a mom for quite a long time.

I had my first of three children over ten years ago now. The fact that I have a ten-year-old child does not really compute in my brain. I am still young, and young people do not have ten year-olds. My next child is eight and the last is five-"and-a-half." But I didn't become a mother ten years ago. I think I became a mom about three or four years ago.

I am reminded just how I felt about motherhood when I see new moms struggling with their babies in slings at the grocery store or pushing their toddlers around in that hellish car-cart that never steers right. My first child stayed in daycare for the first year of his life while I finished a doctoral program in educational administration. I used to rush out of my graduate assistantship, pick him up before his second nap, and whisk him home to snuggle and sleep together. Those afternoons are among my favorite memories.

I defended my dissertation at 8.5 months pregnant with child number two. Who in the world was going to flunk a woman whose belly was visibly crawling during her answers? I passed, graduated, moved home to Mississippi, and Mike started private practice. I assumed I would work at the University and pick up my kids at daycare just like I had before. Life took an unexpected turn.

A few months after being home, Mike's partners broke off to cover a hospital closer to where they lived. All of a sudden, he was the only radiologist in our county hospital. Mike began working 365 days a year, 24 hours a day. Something had to give, and it wasn't Mike's income, so I stayed home with my infant and two-year-old. And I hated it.

I hated several things. First, I hated the long, dull days of sippy cups, diapers, and boring foods. These days seemed like the very longest days on earth. By five-thirty I would start calling Mike, "Are you on your way?" By six I would be banging pots and pans. Second, I hated it when people asked me, "What do you do?" I made up all kinds of answers like "Well, I'm the President of the Public School Foundation," which I was, even though my kids wouldn't be in school for three years, or, "Well, I'm a teacher, but staying with my kids right now."

I knew so many women who sacrificed and scrimped to be able to stay home with their kids, but I was not one of them. I felt selfish for not embracing the opportunity I had. I signed up for every committee and project that came along. I took every Mom and Me class offered, and I put my kids in preschool for half a day.

It took time, experience, and being around some committed

friend-moms to teach me some very important things. First, I didn't understand that mothering can be the most powerful act a woman does. Taking good care of the people we bring into the world may be the most powerful job we are afforded as people—not just women, but as families, aunties, and communities. Mother Theresa famously said, "If you want to change the world, go home and love your family."

For some women, this may mean after work. The critical point is presence. There were many hours I was afforded with my children where I was not fully there. And, there are women who can drop work the minute they walk in the door and give good, quality time to their families.

The other thing I didn't understand was what good care looked like. Good care isn't boring. It is a lot of work—way harder than my doctoral program, probably harder than when I taught 30 alternative school kids in inner city Jackson, Mississippi. It is hard to give good care to kids 24/7. Our daycare workers are the most underpaid, undervalued, *important* professionals in our communities. Good care involves finding good food, fostering health, being present, and creating loving communities.

The last thing I didn't understand was how quickly the time would pass. My three kids are in school now. I am thankful they don't remember when I was filling a role as a mom and not embracing it. They have never had a "stay-at-home-mom" and probably never will. I always have a project or three and a farm.

But what my kids finally have is someone who understands how important it is to be a mother. It is more important than any outside work, project, or role. Taking good care of my kids is at the top of my list now because I understand that while caregiving may be one of the most undervalued roles in our society, society is often wrong.

When people ask what I do now, I am able to say with confidence, "First, I'm a mom." In ten years I have learned that this is an accomplished thing to say.

Caregiving

Caregiving is not necessarily a female job. Aside from breastfeeding, I believe it can be done well by either gender, and by a person who is not the biological parent. Nannies, committed preschool teachers, and extended family are all able to provide good care for children. I believe the problem arises when care is not well-compensated, well-regarded, or well-valued by a culture. And American culture is among the worst when it comes to valuing caregiving in comparison to other developed countries.

Our maternity leaves are shorter, our workdays longer. We don't encourage taking time off to care for children. We penalize people who might have to take off work when their children are sick. And, we are reaping the harvest of children who are raised without valued caregivers.

Remember the pornography statistics from Chapter 3? When do we think those children are viewing pornography on the family computer? When are youth offenders most likely to perpetrate crimes? When are teens most likely to have sex? These events happen most frequently in the 20-25 hours a week between when school is over and when a caregiver gets home, according to the Afterschool Alliance.

While caregiving is undervalued, it is making a comeback, at least in children's early years. *Radical Homemakers* by Shannon Hays describes families who put caregiving at the center of their lives and make sacrifices in order to keep it there as long as possible. Sharing a car, working from home, living with family members to help share the care load are all practices that make radical homemaking possible.

Almost every stay-at-home family I know watches their budget closely to make it happen. They forgo larger homes, lavish vacations, and the newest iPhone. Others weigh the cost of multiple children in day care and decide it doesn't make sense financially.

While financial realities make it impossible for some families to stay home with their children, people are beginning to find creative solutions. I want to see caregiving valued so that our kids think it is just as valid a career as any paid job outside the home. I want to see policies that encourage extended maternal leave. I want teaching preschool to become a coveted position. I want my children to be able to say and do what I could not, proudly claim, "I stay at home with my children." These things can happen when we restore caregiving to the esteemed role it deserves.

Food

One of the biggest things we sacrifice when we do not value caregiving is the food we feed our children. Caregivers were freed from the stove and long production hours of feeding families with the introduction of cheap, processed foods. In my lifetime, the microwave and the Happy Meal both appeared. I remember thinking TV dinners were the most special things with their neat little containers of processed food! However, this ease came with a cost that we didn't foresee.

We are a nation of people who eat, not food, but food-like products full of ingredients we cannot pronounce. I read recently that children today consume more sugar by the time they are eight than people two generations ago consumed in a lifetime. We are overweight, we raise overweight kids, and we are full of food-related illnesses from Crohn's disease to heart failure. We have poisoned our food system, and we are so reliant on a fast, cheap, easy delivery method that we do not care enough to change.

What does food have to do with caregiving? Finding and preparing real food takes time—time we generally don't have when we are working two jobs to pay for our two cars, our larger homes, and our cable bill, or surviving as a single parent. Learning to cook used to happen in families; now, it is an endeavor for adults. I only learned how to cook real food in the last two years. We grew a garden and I realized I had no idea what to do with all the things that came out of it. We ordered a share of a grass-fed cow for the freezer and I had no idea what cuts of meat were prepared which way. We ordered an organic chicken and I had never once dealt with the whole bird.

When we don't value caregiving, we don't value food. Right now we are seeing the epidemics that come from a lack of care about food. Some days I dream of an affordable, organic, drive through dinner option, but most days I realize I have to make food a priority if I want to truly care for my kids.

The way we structure our lives impacts food heavily. My boys play soccer. We spend lots of weekends on the road at tournaments all over the state. Despite the fact that we are at an event celebrating athletes, every field has a little house that feeds the masses of soccer families for the weekend: slushies, soft drinks, hot dogs, pizza, and candy. Every child sports event in town ends with a sugar-filled drink and a sugar-filled snack. Every night the kids have more than two activities means that we eat out. Every birthday is celebrated with cake, ice cream, and a goody bag. Every holiday at school requires junk food. We are up to our eyeballs in crappy food-like substances, and it will take dedicated caregivers who go against this wave of disease to make a difference.

There are some amazing people out there working on these issues. One of my favorite blogs is *100 Days of Real Food* written by a mom who was on a mission to change her kids' food culture. It has loads of practical advice, meal plans, and alternative ideas for snacks and parties. *Wellness Mama* is another blog that provides simple answers for healthier families. *The Sneaky Chef* by Missy Chase Lapine provides simple recipes for disguising healthy foods.

I used this regularly when my kids were smaller. At the preschool my kids attended, parents started a program called "Fresh Start." We got a farmer to bring in one or two local veggies each week, dumped the canned veggies for frozen, and exchanged our healthy snacks for processed food on the menu. We even planted

182

gardens. This was not a government program. It was parents, just like you, who gave a few hours to make health a priority.

What can you do? Pick one thing. Aim to cook four nights a week. The crock pot is my best friend. It doesn't have to be fancy.

Trade sugar for honey in your house. Dump the sodas and juices. If you did no other thing but change your family drink to water, you could probably continue to eat whatever you want and still lose weight, and it would make a huge difference in health and behavior.

Thinking bigger? Tell your sports team to let everyone bring their own snack, and make a list of pro-athlete foods. Ask your child's teacher if you can switch the candy prizes for trinkets. Get a farm-to-school program started in your district. One mom I know started a "snack trade" at school. She brings around healthy snacks and kids actually trade in their Doritos for apples! This is a mom-o-lution, not a school board decision.

Pick your one spot to make change, and go for it.

Health of Young Children

Caregiving takes time. When we are pressed by schedules that are not centered on children's well-being, their health is often compromised. One example is vaccines. My family believes in vaccines. We are thankful that our children won't have to see things like polio or tuberculosis claim their playmates.

We are also skeptical about how many vaccines are required now and how soon they are given to such little bodies. Is a chicken pox vaccine really necessary? What about the roto virus? Given our concerns, we elected to space out our vaccinations. Parents who don't have time to take off work don't have that luxury.

The same goes for the use of antibiotics. When I was still in graduate school with my first child, we gave him that pink ear medicine every other month. We would get rid of his fever and send him back to daycare as quickly as possible. There wasn't time to be sick. Allergy medicine, cough medicine, Tylenol, and baby Ibuprophen all filled our cabinets. At the first sign of an illness, I ran to the doctor to try and get him better quickly.

Our first two kids were so sick so often with ear infections that they both had tubes, and our second had his tonsils out in an excruciating operation at the age of two. By the time our third came around, we had had enough. We kept Cecelia out of daycare for her first year of life, unlike the boys, to try and keep her healthy.

With Cecelia, I was home and more likely to try and take the time to let her immune system kick in on its own. I didn't run for antibiotics quite so quickly or try to get rid of her fevers immediately. I had the time to let her be sick and to heal. More recently, I have begun to focus on building up all three kids' immune systems so that they are more likely to fight off illness and heal quickly. Last time Cecelia got an ear infection, I gave her garlic-filled chicken soup, tons of probiotics, and homeopathy eardrops sold at the drug store. She was fine in a day.

When I was working or in school with children, illness was a stress factor. Now that I am home, I take it as a sign that we need to slow down. I know I am fortunate to have this option. It is an option I think every family should be able to achieve. My friends from Europe say it is expected for a parent to stay home from work until a child is well. If caregiving were valued, I believe it would become a reality for more families.

One of the best resources I can recommend for learning about your kids' immune systems is *The Food Cure for Kids: A Nutritional Approach to Your Child's Wellness.* This is a great book by Natalie Geary, M.D. and Oz Garcia, Ph.D.

I also like *Healing the New Childhood Epidemics: Autism, ADHD, Asthma, and Allergies: The Groundbreaking Program for the 4-A Disorders* by Kenneth Bock.

Another resource that helped me understand how our children's immune system works, even though we did choose spaced vaccinations for our children, was *The Vaccine Illusion* by Tetyana Obukhanych, Ph.D. This author does an amazing job explaining how we can set up our children to best fight infection.

Creating an Ethic of Care

Caregiving is fundamental to healthy people and healthy cultures. Shifting toward a culture that values caregiving takes work, but that work can happen in families. Parents who respect the breadwinner and the caregiver equally send a vitally important message to children. Families who value their preschool teachers enough to fight for increased salaries change things. Extended families who support each other in providing real food, stress relief, and time for healing and recovery from illness model healthy behaviors that will be passed down.

Each of us has a responsibility to develop an Ethic of Care within our families and our communities. Caregiving should be well-compensated, appreciated, and valued. This appreciation of caregiving begins by understanding its real value in terms of health and the real cost associated with its absence.

Section 4

The Wise Elder

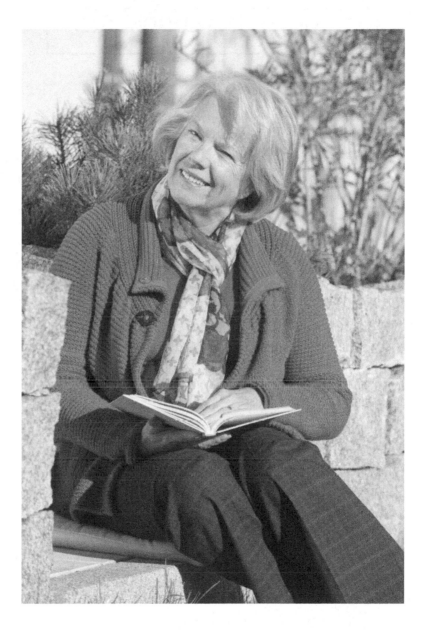

SECTION FOREWORD

"Fleeting?!" responded the tilling man, "Moments? They pass quickly! . . . Why, once a man is finished growing, he still has twenty years of youth. After that, he has twenty years of middle age. Then, unless misfortune strikes, nature gives him twenty thoughtful years of old age. Why do you call that quickly?"
—**Roman Payne**

This section deals with the major physical and psychological challenges women face as they deal with health crises, move through menopause, and begin to focus on overall wellbeing. Some of the things women face as we enter into the Wise Elder years are physical. Others have more to do with how we see and feel about our changing roles.

Female diseases strike many of us by the time we reach this phase of life, and physical, spiritual, and mental health become a primary focus for many women. I also want to note that wisdom is not determined by chronological age. There are some extremely wise young women who, based on life experiences, have much to share with others. For most of us, the learning comes slower, with years of trial and error.

The Wise Elder, or the Crone, represents the wise old woman whose childbearing days are behind her. While history has not been kind to the Crone by picturing her as a witch, our modern understanding of women's wisdom helps us to see her in her full glory. She is compassion and transformation, healing and bawdiness, and death and endings.

She is the respected older woman or grandparent at the heart of the family or community who enjoys life and sharing her experience. Menopause is often associated with the entrance to the Wise Elder years, but despite your age, the Wise Elder archetype may resonate with you if you have gained wisdom, learned from your mistakes, and show a willingness to adapt to changing circumstances, according to *Goddess Guide*.

Entering the Wise Elder years can be a frustrating, negative path for women. Growing older is not always graceful or painless. I believe the way we culturally usher women into the Elder years is important. We want to cultivate Elders who can pass down wisdom and guide younger women.

Remember the epidemic of un-initiated adults mentioned in Chapter 2? So many of us remain stuck in the Maiden and Motherhood roles that the cycle of female development remains incomplete. Wise Elders are the fierce warriors who have nothing to lose and the gentle mentors who have everything to pass on.

What does calling fifty the new thirty or expecting women to remain young-looking in the face and body well into their later years do to our transition into the Elder Years? What expectations for living should we have as we enter our wisdom years? What roles should we play? What dreams should we cultivate as we live longer? What challenges are specific to women in this phase of life?

My own mother and mother-in-law retired this year. I have watched them curiously as they decide how to arrange days that used to be filled with work, meetings, and successful careers.

Suddenly, all the time gifted to them has begun to seem like a burden. They are both avid readers, and my husband's mother loves to travel, but the day-to-day is hard. So much of our identities are wrapped up in what we do for a living or whom we care for. When it comes time to move into the Wise Elder years, some of us flounder as we search for direction. What is our new role? How are we supposed to fill our days meaningfully?

This is also the phase of life when our bodies will no longer be ignored. A lifetime of habits begins to catch up with us. My mother's friend said it was a good thing she retired so she had time to go to all her doctor's appointments. Medications increase, bone density decreases, and aches and pains become routine parts of life. Friends frequently fall victim to one of many female diseases or disorders. Learning to cope with these new realities is not easy.

Oftentimes the Wise Elder years are the first time since Maidenhood that women are afforded time to focus on themselves, but this time with the experience and wisdom gleaned from a lifetime of trial and error. It can be the most creative and fulfilling time of life, but it is also full of health and identity challenges. Coming through these challenges or coping with them gracefully may be the trial-by-fire initiation it takes to become a Wise Elder.

Chapter 11
Female Illnesses

"Having a chronic illness, Molly thought, was like being invaded. Her grandmother back in Michigan used to tell about the day one of their cows got loose and wandered into the parlor, and the awful time they had getting her out. That was exactly what Molly's arthritis was like: as if some big old cow had got into her house and wouldn't go away. It just sat there, taking up space in her life and making everything more difficult, mooing loudly from time to time and making cow pies, and all she could do really was edge around it and put up with it. When other people first became aware of the cow, they expressed concern and anxiety. They suggested strategies for getting the animal out of Molly's parlor: remedies and doctors and procedures, some mainstream and some New Age. They related anecdotes of friends who had removed their own cows in one way or another. But after a while they had exhausted their suggestions. Then they usually began to pretend that the cow wasn't there, and they preferred for Molly to go along with the pretense."   **—Alison Lurie**

Female diseases are not relegated to the Wise Elder years. In fact, women are being diagnosed younger and younger with serious health concerns. However, I placed this chapter in this section of the book because dealing effectively with these diseases and disorders is usually a process that, if we can come through it, or to peace with it, or to terms with it, stands as an initiation rite. Women who have come through the fires of health crisis have valuable wisdom to share with others despite their chronological age.

I want to talk about the Big Ones in women's health: heart disease and cancers. I want to talk about the less "serious," but just as distressing, female diseases like depression and autoimmune diseases, which rob us of quality of life but leave us standing. Sadly, there are too many of these female diseases to recognize in detail here. Please add your story, your struggle, your victories, and your surrenders to the conversation.

What I find encouraging as I delve into the realm of female diseases and disorders, is that women are discovering hope and solutions, and they are compelled to tell their stories of thriving in spite of disease. I found that many women believe these diseases and disorders are preventable and reversible. But what I believe is perhaps the most inspiring is the fortitude of women who do not find answers. Learning to live well in spite of disease and pain is not something Westerners are good at, but I think we are learning.

Women's top five health concerns are heart disease, breast cancer, osteoporosis, depression, and autoimmune diseases, according to D. Zamora, writing for WebMd. Women, along with men, are at risk for cancers, stroke, diabetes, hypertension, and congestive lung failure, but there are certain diseases and disorders that are more prevalent among women. For example, gallstones, irritable bowel syndrome, migraines, urinary tract infections, kidney infections, multiple sclerosis, and rheumatoid arthritis are all more common among women.

In addition to the well know disorders and diseases, women also suffer from a group of "hidden" diseases that are recently gaining much needed attention. Autoimmune diseases are on the rise. CNN did a story on the seven most common "hidden" diseases attacking women's health. They identified polycystic ovary syndrome, fibromyalgia, chronic fatigue syndrome, lupus, multiple sclerosis, rheumatoid arthritis, and irritable bowel syndrome among the secret diseases, according to H. Brown on CNN Health.

Why do these particular diseases manifest in so many women

despite our advanced technologies, screening techniques, and drug therapies? What social stigmas are attached to "female" diseases? Why do we continue to see so many vibrant women brought to their knees by incurable autoimmune disorders? What can we do to create a culture of health, rather than a culture of warriors who must battle disease? What skills and mindsets can we learn that help us live well in the midst of disease and pain that cannot be beaten? These are the questions I think we need to ask as we advocate for health and wellness for all women.

Heart Disease for Women

While surveys show that women are much more concerned about cancer, heart disease demands our attention. Heart disease is the leading cause of death among women but also one of the most preventable. This should not be, ladies. This is one we know how to beat. Diet and lifestyle changes can obliterate this disease. This is one I want to mark off the list for my daughter, and do you know what? We can!

Women's premenopausal levels of estrogen protect us from heart disease. Once these drop post-menopause, our risk increases slightly, but not enough to explain the huge numbers of women who die from heart disease. According to *Harvard Health Publications*, low HDL and high triglycerides are the *only* factors that increase risk of death from heart disease in women over sixty-five. The leading factor for heart attacks in women under the age of sixty-five is metabolic syndrome, which includes large waist size, elevated blood pressure, glucose intolerance, low HDL cholesterol, and high levels of triglycerides. The final factor is smoking. Women who smoke are twice as likely to have a heart attack as men who smoke.

Studies at the Harvard Medical School recommend several diet and lifestyle changes that significantly reduce rates of heart disease. Do not smoke. Even a few cigarettes a day or breathing in second-hand smoke increases your risk for heart disease dramatically. Get thirty minutes or more of exercise. You don't have to go to a gym. Taking the stairs, parking farther away from your workplace, or walking to your job daily are all easy ways to work exercise into your routine. Change your diet. Several crucial ingredients of a heart-healthy diet are whole grains (although those with autoimmune symptoms should avoid wheat and oats), according to the Harvard studies, a variety of fruits and vegetables, nuts (about 5 ounces per week), poly- and monounsaturated fats, fatty fish (such as wild salmon), and limited intake of trans fats.

Reducing stress and treating depression are also among Harvard's top recommendations for preventing heart disease. Stress reduction techniques include exercise, meditation, breathing exercises, and taking steps to remove stressful triggers in your life such as harmful relationships, debt, and over-commitment.

There is some evidence of a two-way relationship between heart disease and depression. According to Dr. Ziegelstein, vice chairman of the Department of Medicine at Johns Hopkins University, "A percentage of people with no history of depression become depressed after a heart attack or after developing heart failure. And people with depression but no previously detected heart disease, seem to develop heart disease at a higher rate than the general population."

Both conventional and alternative medicine seem to agree on important supplements for a healthy heart. Some of these include fish oil, coenzyme Q10, amino acids, and natural extracts like garlic and hawthorn extract. If you are interested in learning more, I suggest Dr. Don Colbert's *The New Bible Cure for Heart Disease: Ancient Truths, Natural Remedies, and the Latest Findings for Your Health Today.* It is a comprehensive guide to all of the most up-to-date research on preventing heart disease.

Heart disease is one of the most solvable conditions women can prevent. I want to share a story by a woman named Deborah, whom I met at a food preservation class. Recently, I read online that due to some health concerns, she was about to make some serious changes in the way she ate. I wrote to her and asked if she would share her story. She was reluctant because, although she had achieved success with weight loss, she hadn't yet been back to the doctor. Finally, she got those results, and this is what she sent me:

> I knew I had some health problems, but my routine checkup in June of this year was a real wake up call. I either needed to make the lifestyle changes I had been talking about for a long time or start taking medications that I really did not want to take. I opted for the lifestyle route. It was NOT easy. No one loves fast food or pasta more than me! But I eliminated all fast food and most processed foods from my diet. I controlled calories but did not go on a super low calorie diet; I focused instead on controlling the amount of carbs and sugar in my diet.
>
> This meant reading every label and investing considerably more time in meal preparation and planning. I began to focus on the quality of the food I was eating and searching out local, fresh options. I found a very helpful blog and cookbook called *The Nourished Kitchen* by Jennifer McGruther.
>
> I searched out healthy options from the local farmer's market and experimented with foods I had never tried before. Meat and vegetables became the mainstay of what I ate, with occasional treats of fresh, local fruit.
>
> Ten weeks later, I feel better. I've lost about 20 pounds. But the real test would be in the next round of blood work. Here's what I found: In ten weeks with these

lifestyle changes I dropped my glucose level by 20 points, my A1C by a full point, my total cholesterol by 108 points, my LDL cholesterol by 60 points, and my triglycerides by 160 points. I still have some health issues that I'm dealing with, but I feel I've made a positive step towards a healthier life.

By sharing her story, Deborah has become a Wise Elder passing on her wisdom. Heart disease does not have to be the number one killer of women. We cure this disease by preventing it. Heart disease is one of the most hopeful diseases out there because, unlike other illnesses, we know exactly what we need to do to avoid it.

That is good news! Culturally, it means a shift. If we know curing the most deadly disease for women requires changing our diet and lifestyle, why do we continue to tolerate food and behaviors we *know* harm ourselves and our daughters? We are addicted to things that are literally killing us.

Here we are, a nation of parents who are fanatical about seat belts as we drive through fast food restaurants for happy meals. We need to look at our behaviors critically and make tough changes. We lead harried and stressful lifestyles (other factors increasing heart disease), which makes it hard to make good dietary choices. What priorities do we need to realign to make healthy choices a reality?

The Big C

While heart disease, lung cancer, and skin cancer pose much more common threats to women, surveys consistently show that females are more concerned with breast and cervical cancers. Theories on the disconnect between fear of risk and realities of risk run the gamut from an overly successful breast cancer awareness campaign to misinformation, or lack of information, the personal fear women have about losing their breasts, or the stigma attached to cancer associated with female anatomy. While all types of cancers strike fear in us, female cancers appear to particularly concern us because they are so connected to our self-image.

Skin cancer is the most common type of cancer among American women. According to the American Cancer Society, it is followed by breast cancer. Breast cancer is the second leading cause of cancer deaths in women, after lung cancer. The five-year relative survival rate for female invasive breast cancer patients has improved from 75 percent in the mid-1970s to 90 percent today. The five-year relative survival rate for women diagnosed with localized breast cancer (disease that hasn't spread to lymph nodes or outside the breast) is 98.5 percent. In cancer that has spread to nearby lymph nodes (regional stage) or to distant lymph nodes or organs (distant stage), the survival rate falls to 84 percent or 24 percent, respectively.

According to the World Health Organization, cervical cancer was once one of the most common causes of cancer death for American women. Over the last 30 years, the cervical cancer death rate has gone down by more than 50 percent. This change is attributed to increased use of the Pap test, a screening procedure that can find changes in the cervix before cancer develops or detect cancer early in its most curable stage.

For breast cancer, the disease can be detected in its early stages through breast self-examination, clinical breast examination, and mammography screening. In general, however, mammography screening has led to a substantial reduction—estimated to be about 15 percent—in breast cancer mortality.

The debates surrounding female cancer detection and treatment are in full swing. On one end of the spectrum, doctors and cancer advocacy groups tout early detection through self-exams, mammograms, and Pap tests as the key components in battling these diseases successfully. My husband is a radiologist who comes home at least once a month depressed because of a mammogram that he knows shows a cancer that has gone too far. He says repeatedly, "If she had just come in a year ago…"

On the other end, studies continue to provide mixed results about diagnostic efficacy. The hypothesis that screening is vital to health and longevity is being turned on its head, with researchers asserting that mammograms and Pap smears can cause more harm than good for women of certain ages, according to K. Sack writing in the *New York Times*. It is hard to follow the arguments that say these studies are a ploy for insurance companies to pay for less wellness visits versus those who believe the diagnostics are truly harmful. For those of us who grew up with pink ribbons stuck on everything from t-shirts to fruit, this recent debate is confusing. The best short article I can recommend to summarize the information clearly, comes from Peggy Orenstein and is entitled "Our Feel Good War On Breast Cancer."

Researching cancer in general for this section proved to be the most frustrating subject of this book. Try Googling "Are cancer rates increasing or decreasing?" The conflicting information is baffling. Cancer, it appears, is all over the board. Some types of cancers are decreasing in incidence, while others are on the rise.

Advanced technology and diagnostic tools may account for the increase more than actual rates of incidence. Treatments for cancer, however, appear promising. According to the American Cancer Society, the cancer death rate for men and women combined fell 20 percent from its peak in 1991 to 2010, the most recent year for which data is available.

Medical treatments for cancer are advancing rapidly. While surgeries, chemotherapy, radiation therapy, and targeted drug therapy top the list as the most common types of cancer treatments, new therapies are being tested all the time. Immunotherapy, hyperthermia, stem cell transplants, hormonal blockers, and photodynamic therapies are among those being studied as effective treatments, according to cancer.org.

There is also a growing body of evidence that lifestyle changes improve cancer survival rates. A pair of Yale Cancer Center interventional studies involving breast cancer survivors found that lifestyle changes in the form of healthy eating and regular exercise can decrease biomarkers related to breast cancer recurrence and mortality.

Alternative therapies abound when it comes to preventing and treating cancer. When I spoke with cancer survivors about any alternative therapies they encountered on their journeys, many of them recommended one book, *Radical Remissions* by Dr. Kelly Turner. Turner defines "radical remission" as any cancer remission that is statistically unexpected ... and occurs whenever:

- a person's cancer goes away without using any conventional medicine; or

- a cancer patient tries conventional medicine, but the cancer does not go into remission, so he or she switches to alternative methods of healing, which do lead to a remission; or

- V. Agnew offers a third definition: When a cancer patient uses conventional medicine and alternative healing methods at the same time in order to outlive a statistically dire prognosis (i.e., an cancer with less than 20 percent chance of five-year survival).

During the study, Turner identified more than seventy-five methods that cancer survivors said they used as a part of their healing journeys. Nine of these methods were used by almost every one of them.

They are: radically changing your diet, taking control of your health, following your intuition, using herbs and supplements, increasing positive emotions, embracing social support, deepening your spiritual connection, and having strong reasons for living. The following excerpt is by Sandra Bender, who has been in remission for almost a decade using *Radical Remissions* as a guide:

When I read *Radical Remissions* I realized I am a radical survivor. After my sixth chemotherapy treatment and two second opinions I asked my oncologist whether she thought my cancer could be cured. She said, "No." So I asked whether she thought I would die from this cancer, and she said, "Yes." She was not being unkind. She told me the truth only after I asked.

When we settled in the car for the drive home, my husband Nate reached out his hand and said, "I want us to agree that we will not stop until your cancer is cured." I squeezed his hand in agreement. Those were the most loving, hopeful, healing words he could have said.

I was on my own to find treatment [that is] more hopeful than conventional chemotherapy. Through talking with friends and family I learned about a treatment center that integrates nutrition, supplements, physical therapy, massage, counseling, and yoga with standard chemotherapy. I believe as a result of integrative cancer therapy, I have been in remission for eight years and still counting. The most difficult part was to realize I had to make my own decisions about treatment instead of relying on conventional doctors.

Women supporting women through cancer seems to be one of our greatest achievements, culturally. We successfully took a silent killer and, in two generations, turned it into a public campaign that is universally recognized. Cancer, even female cancer, is no longer shameful. Brave women are telling their stories of survival and demanding new research and better answers.

Cancer treatments and diagnostics continue to improve following these calls for action. Functional medicine offers women real hope. Spiritual, emotional, and lifestyle changes enhance chances of success. And, similar to other female diseases I have covered, women are getting much of their information from shared stories by other women.

Depression

Depression is a whole other book. It is that dark shadow that plagues nearly all of us at some point in our lives, but for many women, depression is a slignificant health factor. Major depression is the leading cause of disability for Americans between the ages of 15 and 44, according to the CDC, and among the top five health concerns for women. And, according to the National Institute of Mental Health (NIMH), the largest scientific organization dedicated to mental health issues, women are 70 percent more likely than men to experience depression during the course of their lifetimes.

Importantly, depressive disorders are associated with increased prevalence of chronic diseases, according to an article written by Chapman, Perry and Strine on the CDC website. Depressive disorders can precipitate chronic disease, and chronic disease can make symptoms of depression worse. Depressive disorders and chronic disease are interrelated, a factor which has important implications for both chronic disease management and the treatment of depression.

Antidepressants have become a first line of defense against depression. According to the CDC, antidepressants were the third most common prescription drug taken by Americans of all ages in 2005–2008 and the most frequently used by persons aged 18–44 years.

From 1988–1994 through 2005–2008, the rate of antidepressant use in the United States among all ages increased nearly 400 percent. It has since leveled off. That is a lot of antidepressants; although, as discussed earlier, depression is only one of the reasons doctors describe antidepressants. Women suffering from PMS and autoimmune disorders are also commonly prescribed antidepressant medications.

While antidepressants are effective for many women, they do not address underlying issues that may cause depression, and there is little discussion of long-term side effects. Dr. Kelly Brogan, "I see mental illness and I think of a gene/environment mismatch—I look to sources of inflammation and hormonal disruption, such as diet, stress, sedentary lifestyle, and toxic exposures, and I get to the root." If you are interested in learning more about getting to root causes, I recommend *Treating Depression Naturally* by Joan Mathews Larsons and *Unstuck: Your Guide to the Seven Stage Journey Out of Depression* by James S. Gordon, M.D.

If you are interested in learning more about the long-term side effects of antidepressants, I recommend Peter Breggin's landmark article "Brain Disabling Treatments in Psychiatry" and Grace Jackson's book, *Rethinking Psychiatric Drugs* as resources.

One of the most troubling side effects of antidepressants is getting off of them or "tapering." Few of us are told about the harsh realities of coming off a medication when we fill our first prescription. Dr. Kelly Brogan writes: "I work to restore resiliency prior to taper by unearthing physiologic imbalances, autoimmune phenomenon, and perceived stress before medication decreases as a means of mitigating the taper's effects—helping the body to become more adaptive to the absence of medication because it has more available resources in wellness. However, there is no antidote, no magic bullet, when patients are in the throes [sic] of taper. This is why the informed consent process becomes paramount. Patients need to know, before filling that first prescription, that their episode is likely to resolve on its own within three months (no treatment), that there are effective alternatives, and that there are significant potential short and long term risks."

While I do believe that there is a time and a place for antidepressants, I think it is important to understand that there are other ways to overcome one of the main health concerns for women. If you are not in a place to deal with underlying causes, by all means, take your meds. Depression is real, and it takes a lot of hard work to come through it. Medications can be helpful in mitigating the effects, but they do not cure the cause. Many people, including myself, have become reliant on the medication just to survive.

I took antidepressants for fifteen years. Every time I went off, I crashed. It was not until I began to look at the underlying causes of my depression that I found the tools needed to begin to heal them. If you do not change the system that fosters depression, there is no way to live without the medication.

I found several natural medications that were every bit as effective as the pharmaceutical ones, except that they do not have the long-term or short-term side effects, such as St. John's Wort and amino acids. I eat a pretty strict paleo diet, because I know what gluten and sugar do to my mood. I meditate every day, and I take the amino acid SAM-e every day, just like I took my Effexor or Prozac. It makes me methylate (I have no real understanding of what this means in biological terms, but it works).

The difference is, the amino acid addresses the process that enables my body to make the correct chemical, rather than just putting those chemicals directly into my system. It also allows me to feel fully. It takes all these things for me to be off meds. It's like a part-time job with a lot of hours, but for me, it is worth it.

I used to think women who went off medication could not have been as bad off as I was. I just assumed I would be on medication the rest of my life. I was wrong. I like being able to feel life's ups and downs without sinking.

I like being a little bit "uncomfortably un-numb" since I have learned tools that allow me to be my own life preserver. Taking the magic bullet route is what we have become used to. Medications for ADHD, depression, anxiety, and weight loss all come with a hidden price tag.

I urge you to look into long-term solutions for yourselves and your families. There is usually a way to free oneself from the medication treadmill. It is not quick or easy, but it might be worth it.

Moving into wiser years requires that we take a look at our demons, rather than sweeping them under the rug. Facing root causes of depression and learning to live peacefully with our range of emotions is something Wise Elders know how to do. It is one of the most concrete gifts they can pass on to younger generations. Wise Elders guided me out of my dependence on medication to deal with my emotions through writing, conversation, and good work. I found them in books, over cups of tea, in my community, and at church. These women had learned how to bring life into balance, and I learned from them. It takes practice and the right tools to be able to learn to live with a wide range of feelings. One of my biggest breakthroughs was figuring out that it is not normal to feel good all the time. Feeling okay is, sometimes, okay.

Autoimmune Disorders

Autoimmune disorders are some of the most common diseases among females, but also among the most misunderstood. There are almost 100 different autoimmune disorders, and symptoms vary. Usually, people go in for tests when they suffer over a long period of time with fatigue, depression, or generalized pain.

Rheumatoid arthritis, type 1 diabetes, psoriasis, alopecia, lupus, thyroid disease, Addison's disease, pernicious anemia, celiac disease, multiple sclerosis, myasthenia gravis, autoimmune hepatitis, and Guillain-Barre syndrome are just a few of the ailments that scientists now think stem from a common phenomenon: the activation of the body's immune system against the body itself.

Researchers are beginning to add conditions like Parkinson's, Alzheimer's, and even ADHD to this category. Chronic fatigue syndrome and fibromyalgia are also classified in this category.

The National Institute of Health estimates that five to eight percent of Americans have an autoimmune disorder; it is much more common among females. Depending on the definition, I have seen rates as high as one in twelve people, and one in nine females. According to the national Institutes of Health, the causes of autoimmune disorders are associated with viruses, infections, genetics, and environmental factors. They often appear in groups, and symptoms often continue throughout a person's life. Although the causes are not fully understood, autoimmune disorders cause the immune system to attack healthy tissue.

While autoimmune disorders are not curable, the goals of treatment are to reduce symptoms, control the autoimmune process, and maintain the body's ability to fight disease. Treatments include supplements to replace a substance the body lacks, such as thyroid hormone, vitamin B12, or insulin. Blood transfusions are used if blood is affected, and physical therapy is used to help with bones, joints, and muscles. According to the National Institutes of Health, there are immunosuppressive medicines available to decrease the body's immune system response, such as prednisone.

What is so frustrating about autoimmune disorders is their lack of specificity. People usually go to multiple doctors to receive a diagnosis, and once they finally do receive a diagnosis, treatment options are not always effective. The side effects alone are often miserable. Autoimmune disorders are some of the most frustrating diseases, and they are increasing in incidence.

There are many theories as to why this is happening. One theory that makes a lot of sense to me is our "war on bacteria." We live in the age of the hand-sanitizers, pasteurized and radiated food, and over-prescribed antibiotics.

While we have ended many of the heartbreaking bacterial diseases in our culture, we may be going too far. There are a whole lot of bacteria that protect us from the small percentage of bad bacteria. If we kill off all bacteria, our immune systems may become confused. For a great article on this topic, check out "Dirtying Up Our Diets" by Jeff Leach.

Food and health writer Michael Pollan explains how beneficial microbes impact our immune systems by helping them to distinguish between good and bad. Some researchers believe that the alarming increase in autoimmune diseases in the West may be linked to a disruption in the ancient relationship between our bodies and their "old friends" — the microbial symbionts with whom we coevolved.

"These claims sound extravagant, and in fact many microbiome researchers are careful not to make the mistake that scientists working on the human genome did a decade or so ago, when they promised they were on the trail of cures to many diseases," writes Pollan. "We're still waiting. Yet whether any cures emerge from the exploration of the second genome, the implications of what has already been learned—for our sense of self, for our definition of health, and for our attitude toward bacteria in general—are difficult to overstate."

Pollan believes health should "be thought of as a collective property of the human-associated microbiota, as one group of researchers recently concluded in a landmark review article on microbial ecology—that is, as a function of the community, not the individual."

"Such a paradigm shift comes not a moment too soon, because as a civilization, we've just spent the better part of a century doing our unwitting best to wreck the human-associated microbiota with a multi-fronted war on bacteria and a diet notably detrimental to its well-being," continues Pollan. "Researchers now speak of an impoverished 'Westernized microbiome' and ask whether the time has come to embark on a project of "restoration ecology" — not in the rain forest or on the prairie but right here at home, in the human gut."

What does this mean for autoimmune disorders and treatments? What behaviors can we change or control that might lessen our chances of developing one of these life-altering problems? What practices could we employ to help our kids' chances of developing a healthy immune response? Of course, some of the autoimmune puzzle is in our genes, but what about the rest of it?

When I was researching the latest on autoimmune success stories, I found a couple of great books and blogs I want to share with you. *Alternative autoimmune: Wellness in a whole new light* is a good blog that shares success stories, practical tips, and resources for people suffering from all kinds of autoimmune disorder.

The author herself spent ten years trying to get the bottom of her own diagnosis. She also does health coaching via Skype. *Paleo Magazine* hosts an entire page devoted to autoimmune bloggers on its site.

Mary Shoman's *Living Well with Autoimmune Disease* is a great place to start for thorough coverage of all standard treatments, but it is also a comprehensive guide to alternative treatments. I highly recommend the book *The Autoimmune Epidemic* by Donna Jackson Nakazawa.

This investigative journalist is relentless in her search for answers about why this group of diseases is reaching epidemic proportions. Finally, I recommend checking out *The Immune System Recovery Plan* website. The website provides a step-by-step plan by Susan Blum, M.D. for healing your immune system.

The most compelling formula for health, I believe, comes from physician Terry Wahls who was diagnosed with multiple sclerosis in 2002. If you watch one video on autoimmune diseases, Google hers: *How I Went From Wheelchair To Walking By Changing My Diet*. Her formula is simple and effective. It has changed the way she practices medicine and does research, but most importantly it has impacted her quality of life.

The good news is that people are finding lifestyle solutions that mitigate the effects of these diseases. In my research, I found more success stories than I ever expected. More good news comes from the medical front. Scientists are learning how to "switch off" autoimmune diseases. Autoimmune diseases are baffling and debilitating, but determined individuals and dedicated science are making a dent in them. However, finding a cure is not the only road to living well with autoimmune diseases.

I love this blog post by Sarah Wilson as she comments on an article by Meghan O'Rourke in the *New Yorker*:

> **Like me, O'Rourke reaches a point where she's largely able to manage her disease through diet—no gluten, no sugar, meditation, kefir, avoiding nightshades, etc. etc. I've tried it all. And it's all required to maintain something resembling a normal life when you have a tricky AI.**
>
> **But, and these are the two points of note: She hasn't been cured as such. The "flares" and cycles continue. Her focus on trying to find a cure, and on controlling the AI, has seen her AI control her. Her A-ha moment comes, however, when her endocrinologist delivers blunt news after a "lapse."**
>
> **Despite her best efforts to control things with her lifestyle habits, she seems to go backwards, causing her to lament, again, that no one knows what the hell is going on. Says the endocrinologist to O'Rourke: "This may just be how it's going to be. You may always feel like you're eighty percent."**
>
> **Wow. And shit. And tears. And just for good measure, let's read that again: You may always feel like you're eighty percent.**

While I think it is safe to say medical and alternative treatments do exist to help mitigate the effects of autoimmune diseases, it is also safe to say that learning to live peaceably with these lifelong disorders is important.

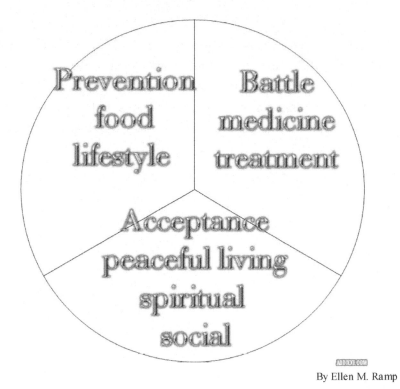

By Ellen M. Ramp

In fact, it may be the key to living well with this group of diseases that do not have a cure and continue to become more common. Tara Brach is the landmark author on living well with pain. I recommend her books *Radical Acceptance,* and *True Refuge* as great places to start.

Heart disease, cancer, depression, and autoimmune disorders are realities for most women at some point in our lives. Learning not only to survive these diseases but also to thrive in spite of them is a great challenge. Thankfully, science is making progress in effectively dealing with these diseases. Natural alternatives are becoming more readily available.

More importantly, we are beginning to understand what it takes to foster a culture of wellness, rather than one that constantly battles disease. The wisdom gained as women move through these challenges with resolve is one of the most valuable tools we can pass on to younger women.

Wise Elders lead us toward balance. I have watched my own mother gracefully and powerfully learn to live well in spite of Parkinson's disease while writing this book. Her balance of courage and acceptance inspires me. She demonstrates daily that the disease does not define your essence. We are all body, mind, and spirit.

Chapter 12
Premenopause & Perimenopause

"The first indication of menopause is a broken thermostat. It's either that or your weight. In any case, if you don't do something, you could be dead by August."
—**Dorothea Benton Frank**

As a young teacher, and now as a parent, I always wished school started at nine in the morning to match children's schedules better (and mine, for that matter). I was always told school schedules were set by menopausal women who got too hot to teach late into the afternoon and who were up early from night sweats by five in the morning.

Then there was the scene in *Fried Green Tomatoes* where a mild-mannered Southern woman turned into menopausal Towanda and smashed into a younger girl's car on purpose when she cut her off in a parking lot. That is about the extent of what I knew about menopause until last year.

Let me tell you how surprised I was to learn that I am in a menopause category. Pre-menopause is something I had not heard of until my last gynecological visit. I was just in my childbearing years four years ago, and already they are talking about menopause? It feels all too fast for me!

One of my closest friends is about ten years older than I am, and she is in the throes of true perimenopause right now. She is one of the most competent, least complaining, toughest people I know, and menopause has thrown her for a loop in the last year. This scares me!

Given my history, the odds are that menopause won't be a pretty ride. Is it for any woman? Are there women out there who sail through the transition into wise womanhood? Is it possible to navigate the waters of "The Change" without synthetic hormones?

Once the change is done, are we free? I cannot speak from experience on this topic, but I will share what I am finding out.

Premenopause or Perimenopause
Or What We Call Plain Menopause

I remember my own even-keeled mother doing some totally out of character things like going up to a bunch of teenaged boys in a hotel we were staying in and explaining to them exactly how much noise they were making. My brother and I wondered, *What's wrong with mom?* At some point, perimenopause symptoms seem to hijack most women's bodies.

Perimenopause (I have to laugh because this word does not exist in my computer's spellcheck) includes the period of time a woman's body transitions toward permanent infertility (menopause). My goodness! That sounds drastic—permanent infertility.

I have seen ages anywhere from 30-50 describing this stage. Mayo Clinic says that the level of your estrogen rises and falls unevenly during perimenopause and the length of your menstrual cycles begins to vary. Once you have gone through twelve consecutive months without a menstrual period, you have officially reached menopause.

The symptoms can be troubling, as they have been for my friend. She says it started with weight gain, spread to an overall feeling that her body just didn't feel right, and is manifesting itself currently with temperature and mood swings. Mayo Clinic lists these symptoms: menstrual irregularity, hot flashes and sleep problems, mood changes, vaginal and bladder problems, changes in sexual function, decreased fertility, and changes in cholesterol.

Another common factor associated with menopause is osteoporosis. Osteoporosis, or thinning bones, can result in painful fractures. According to the National Osteoporosis Foundation, almost half of all post-menopausal women will suffer from a bone fracture because of osteoporosis. Risk factors for osteoporosis include aging, being female, low body weight, low sex hormones or menopause, smoking, and some medications.

Perimenopause sounds like a scene in one of my boys' sci-fi movies where the spacecraft careens out of control and lands on an alien planet.

Why is the natural aging process so rough on women's bodies? What can we do to alleviate some of this turbulence, and do symptoms have to be so exasperating? Is there a better way to move into the post-reproductive years? I want to discuss some of these issues in this chapter.

Treatments for Perimenopause

Formerly, all perimenopausal women were prescribed Menopausal Hormone Therapy (MHT), which was previously called Hormone Replacement Therapy. I thought it was generally understood today that MHT was not a good option. However, some women do use menopausal hormone therapy (MHT) to help control the symptoms of menopause. MHT involves taking the hormones estrogen and progesterone. Women who no longer have a uterus take just estrogen.

MHT can be very good at helping with moderate to severe symptoms of the menopausal transition and preventing bone loss, but MHT also has some risks, especially if used for a long time, according to the National Cancer Institute. MHT can help menopause by reducing hot flashes, night sweats, poor sleep, and irritability. It can treat vaginal discomfort and pain during sex. MHT slows bone loss and eases mood swings and depressive symptoms. However, for some women, MHT may increase their chances of blood clots, heart attack, stroke, breast cancer, and gall bladder disease.

When I read this I thought, what is the big deal? We generally ignore "possible risks." Think about the drug commercials with their ridiculously long caveats at the end. Drug companies spend billions on advertising, and even as they state these risks out loud and at a very fast clip, we believe they are safe because our government agency approves them.

If you only read the government agency's statement about MHTs, you would probably come to the conclusion that, like anything, there are risks, but the benefits are greater. It takes digging a little deeper to find the truth.

The National Cancer Institute produces a fact sheet full of studies on MHTs and studies regarding safety. Research from the WHI studies has shown that MHT is associated with the following harms: urinary incontinence, dementia, stroke, blood clots, heart attack, breast cancer, and lung cancer.

There are some disturbing facts in this study. Statistics on dementia alone are enough to cause concern, and it is fairly easy to deduce that MHT causes cancers to grow more quickly. I am not generally a conspiracy theorist, but … this does not look good!

A Brief History of Hormone Treatment describes a big push by pharmaceuticals to keep women forever young. In the decades between the 1966 book *Feminine Forever,* which touted the positive benefits of hormone replacement therapy (later the author was accused by his own son of being paid by the drug company that made estrogen), and the 2002 Women's Health Initiative (WHI) study. It explains how hormone treatment became the most prescribed drug in the country.

The WHI study revealed evidence that taking hormones did not protect healthy women against heart disease and stroke. It was the WHI study that showed that women who took the combination of estrogen and progestin had increased their risk for breast cancer, stroke, heart attack, and blood clots.

So What Are Women to Do?

Even if you decide that you will not subject your body to the science experiment of synthetically made hormones, there is still the maddening roller coaster of menopause to deal with. What are some safe, effective approaches to dealing with perimenopause and all its gory symptoms?

The best advice I can add to the dialogue at this point is to read two books. Dr. John Lee writes the *What Your Doctor May Not Tell You About...* series. The first book is on premenopause and the second is on menopause.

I read both, and they give very similar advice. Both books promote natural progesterone as part of the solution. The difference between natural and synthetic hormones is explained in detail. Apparently your body has a much easier time assimilating natural, animal, and plant derived hormones than it does chemically produced hormones. These books are comprehensive, and I like that they include the spiritual and emotional components of this phase of life. They also emphasize the necessary diet and supplement regimens to follow to support your body through perimenopause and beyond.

The aforementioned diet and lifestyle improvements are central to dealing successfully with perimenopause. Cutting out the inferior foods and increasing the good ones is as important a step as taking any medication. Maintaining steady glucose levels and decreasing stress with exercise, prayer, or meditation are all equally important. Many women get help from functional medicine practitioners, acupuncturists, and Traditional Chinese Medicine. Osteoporosis associated with menopause can be significantly mitigated by getting enough calcium and vitamin D and by quitting smoking and by performing weight bearing exercises regularly, according to the National Osteoporosis Foundation.

Balancing your hormones naturally is possible. According to A. Shah, writing for mindbodygreen.com, some of the recommendations include cutting carbohydrates, supplementing with omega-3s, avoiding commercial oils, cutting caffeine, and adding coconut and avocado oils. Other recommendations are adding vitamin D, trying maca root or chaste tree, getting rid of hormone disruptors in your home (household cleaners and personal care products with parabens, phthalates, or bisphenol-A), and managing stress with meditation and exercise.

Return to Rites of Passage

Menopause has been associated with drying up, losing the life-giving force, and, more optimistically, being freed from the burden of child production. It is seldom valued in our culture as a transition to the Wise Elder. What if we took all that negativity that surrounds menopause and turned it into the last quest women have to adventure on before they become trusted elders of their communities?

I know it is a bit much for our current framework, but how many wise premenopausal women do you know? Is there a chance we could embrace this transition as the most formidable and important on our journeys? Or am I just projecting wishful thinking on my uncertain menopausal future?

I don't think I am deluding myself. In many cultures throughout history, menopause was—and in some places still is—an honored rite of passage. I came across this Chinese understanding of menopause by J. Griffen in *The Spirit of Maat*: "According to traditional Chinese medicine, during menopause there is a natural decline in what's known as 'Precious Essence'—which is a 'yin,' or passive feminine energy. But while Precious Essence declines, Chinese medicine also sees a corresponding increase in 'yang' energy, or active masculine energy. That increase is an important part of the change that's happening. In this view, menopause can be a time of life when many women move from being passive to setting boundaries and becoming more goal oriented."

Many women learn to speak their minds more easily. Women change. Their personalities change, their outlook on life changes. This is part of the process. This can be a rich time, and deep inward direction can come out of it."

Just as I would like to reframe coming into menstruation with reverence, I believe we can do the same for the transition out of it. Creating a rite of passage around menopause refashions the whole experience. Living at odds with our natural cycles of femininity is not working. It doesn't make the cramps or the mood swings or the hot flashes budge no matter how strongly we hate them.

What if mind over matter is one of the keys to successfully transitioning into the Wise Elder years? What if we trick ourselves into believing these pains are powerful? What if believing they are powerful transforms them from something ugly and unpleasant into something sacred?

The other resource at the top of my list for perimenopause is writer and teacher Susun Weed, whom I have quoted at length. She is my hero when it comes to understanding women's passages through life. She has beautiful and practical books, CDs, online courses, and blogs on all manner of what she calls "Wise Woman Ways." Even if you choose not to incorporate herbalism into your health regime, her re-sculpted vision of menopause is worth reading.

Menopausal Years, the Wise Woman Way
By Susun Weed

Menopause is a period of transition and metamorphosis, like puberty. It consists of three stages: isolation, melt down, and emergence. Each stage calls forth new energies and new perceptions of our selves. Each stage has different demands, different tasks, and different needs.

Wise Woman Ways, such as simple ceremony, compassionate self-care, and daily use of dooryard plants, can be of tremendous benefit to women going through menopause. Please allow me to share with you some of my favorite herbs for easing hot flashes, sleeplessness, and other distresses of The Change. They're easy to find; you may already know them as weeds! These plants, and their cautions and contraindications, are described in detail in my book *Menopausal Years, The Wise Woman Way*. Please refer to it before you decide whether or not to use any of these green allies to aid you during your menopausal years.

Calcium intake during and after menopause must be high to maintain health. But calcium in pills can't compare to calcium in plants when it comes to maintaining healthy, flexible bones. Bones are made of a dozen minerals besides calcium (potassium, manganese, magnesium, silica, iron, zinc, selenium, boron, phosphorus, sulphur, and chromium), all of which are found in rich supply in the roots and leaves of edible weeds and herbs. Eating weeds is my preferred way of preventing osteoporosis and insuring freedom from heart disease, depression, headaches, leg cramps, and joint pain.

There are scores of calcium/mineral-rich plants to choose from, such as the aromatic leaves of sage, peppermint, lemon balm, bergamot, rosemary, and thyme; the cooked or fresh greens of lamb's quarters, amaranth, dandelion, chicory, comfrey, stinging nettle, chickweed, parsley, watercress, kale, collards, and cabbage; the flowers of red clover; and the roots of yellow dock, dandelion, chicory, and burdock. For maximum extraction of mineral richness, I cook with these herbs, drink them as infusions, and steep them in vinegar.

Seaweeds have incredibly generous amounts of calcium and minerals, too. I make it a practice to eat seaweeds such as kelp, dulse, and nori daily, as condiments, and a seaweed such as wakame,

218

hijiki, arame, and kombu once a week, cooked with carrots or in a soup.

Hormones are a hot topic for menopausal women. To help myself with hormonal surges and drops, I prefer to use tinctures of plants rich in plant hormones (phytosterols) rather than prescribed hormones (estrogen replacement or hormone replacement), which actually elevate the risk of heart disease and osteoporosis, contrary to advertising, and are linked to increases in breast and uterine cancers. Women whose blood is rich in plant hormones have the lowest rates of cancer in the world. Plants rich in phytosterols include: roots of dong quai, ginseng, wild yam, black cohosh, black haw, dandelion; flowers of hops, yarrow, red clover; leaves of stinging nettle, sage; berries/seeds/hips of chaste tree/vitex, fenugreek, roses.

Favorite herbs for menopausal women:

Oatstraw infusion (Avena sativa) strengthens the nerves, helps reduce emotion distress, promotes sound sleep, keeps the bones and heart strong, and strengthens libido. The tincture is a stronger sedative but not nourishing to the bones and heart. Oats for breakfast is an excellent way to "take" this herb, but avoid pills and capsules. Oatstraw baths are exceptionally calming. Instructions for making one are in my green book: *Healing Wise.*

Nettle infusion (Urtica dioica) strengthens the adrenals, eases anxiety, increases energy, helps prevent night sweats, builds blood, protects bones and heart. Eating cooked nettle is another excellent way to gather its benefits, as is nettle vinegar. I avoid freeze-dried, encapsulated, or tinctured nettle, believing all these forms ineffective and over-priced.

Motherwort (Leonurus)—tincture of the fresh flowering tops— is a favorite with menopausal women, their daughters and their mothers. A few drops (up to 25 at a time) will calm emotions, relieve heart palpitations (and strengthen the heart), reduce the severity of hot flashes, increase vaginal lubrication, moderate and eliminate PMS and menstrual cramping. Motherwort vinegar is a fantastic tonic, and tasty, thank goodness. The tea is violently bitter and disliked by 99 out of 100 women, including me, yuck.

Dandelion (Taraxacum)—any part, in any form—is a superb strengthener for the liver, the control center for hot flashes. Dandelion improves digestion, especially of calcium, helps relieve headaches, and sees to it that the liver provides steady blood sugar supplies. Dandelion wine (from the blossoms) is the most elegant way to take this remedy, but the cooked leaves and vinegars (as well as the pickled parts) of the roots and/or leaves are also excellent nourishing digestives. The tincture, especially of the root, is considered the strongest medicine, but doesn't contain bone-building nutrients, so is less ideal than the other forms.

Startling facts about menopause: The Grandmother Hypothesis maintains that "menopause, like a big brain and an upright posture, is one of the essential traits of the human which allowed us to colonize the world."

Menopause is not a recent phenomenon, but an ancient women's mystery, with special gifts for the woman who uses its energies wisely. Estrogen is not one hormone, but many, and our bodies continue to make estrogens all of our lives. The adrenals, the fat tissues, and perhaps the uterus make estrogens.

The levels of hormones in a woman's blood are never higher than when she is in menopause.

Herbal hormones (phytosterols, or phytoestrogens) are usable by the body and, in contrast to prescribed hormones, protect against breast cancer. " *Reprinted with permission*

* * *

Reframing the way we view The Change of life, valuing what Wise Elders have to offer communities, and discovering effective ways to usher women successfully through menopause are important steps in creating initiated adults who can help guide younger generations.

For further reading, I recommend Jennifer Boire's *The Tao of Turning 50: What Every Woman in her 40s Needs to Know.* Boire writes, "Look beyond the symptoms and reframe the experience as a rite of passage. Recognize these symptoms are labor pains. You are in a major phase of initiation into a new Self. All you hear about is hot flashes and night sweats. But menopause is a transition worthy of ritual and self-care; you are worthy of attending to yourself with loving kindness and compassion."

Finding healthy solutions to mitigate physical symptoms and reshaping menopause into an honored rite of passage to mitigate emotional ones are important steps for women. We are beginning to move in the right direction by looking for medical solutions that do not have long-term, harmful effects on women.

The next step is embracing menopause as a powerful and necessary shift into a new phase of living. Boire concludes, "The good news is that you will resurface; you will find yourself again in the second half of life. You will come through this rite of passage with greater self-confidence, a sense of maturity and the courage to find your voice. The post menopausal woman is the Wise Woman, the one who gives us all a survival edge."

Chapter 13

Wise Elder Advice on Living

"She was a woman who knew who she was and how she had gotten there."
—*Lisa Mangum*

For this chapter, I invited three Wise Elders from my community to share advice on living as a woman. These women stood out immediately in my mind when I thought:

Who are the Wise Elders in my world?

Two are mothers to actual children. One is a mother to simple, revolutionary ideas. All are mothers to our community and usher younger women into wiser ways of living either by example or through caring nurture, or both. These women popped into my mind reflexively because of their grace in adversity, their trueness to themselves, and the impact they have had on those around them. They are Steel Magnolias for certain: tough, tender, and open.

Here is their wisdom.

Elizabeth Hawkins

Elizabeth has been retired for thirteen years, pursuing interests she never had time for during her working years. During those thirteen years she has been widowed and is now remarried. Elizabeth reunited with a high school beau, and the two of them spend time with their children and grandchildren, and travel in their RV. They are busy with other interests including participating in two orchestras, two choruses, and two theatres; playing bridge and cooking. Elizabeth's career began as an English teacher and transitioned to university research administration, which led her to continue her studies through a doctoral degree. She has also served her church for over thirty years as pianist.

222

While Elizabeth is obviously accomplished and leads a full, busy life, I didn't ask her to share her advice because of those traits. I asked her to share her advice because she is a child of the segregated Mississippi Delta who goes to Buddhist Retreats, teaches Sunday School, and has survived adversity with more beauty, confidence, and grace than any woman I know. Here is what she had to say about womanhood:

* * *

I'm not sure that I can change a culture that puts so much emphasis on sex and physical beauty. Girls must grow up in a personal world that reinforces their value as total human beings. Beauty is far more than measurements, skin type, and hair color. It is self-confidence, self-reliance, knowledge, developed talents, and a personality that is loving and kind. As women, we can influence our own homes and our smaller communities within the culture at large—church, school, social and civic organizations—so that our sons and daughters grow up with healthy attitudes about other human beings and their relationships to them.

I think my advice to my teenaged self would closely follow my mother's example and advice. She emphasized healthful eating, good personal care, and strong self-image. Her comment when I went out was always, "Remember who you are." In retrospect, I realize that her emphasis on valuing myself played a large part in helping me to develop healthy relationships and goals for my life. In addition, I would encourage my teenaged self to talk about my feelings, emotional and physical, and the ethical tensions that occur when societal influences conflict with values taught at home.

Taking care of young children is the most rewarding and the most exhausting job in the world! My advice is to find time alone with each child daily, if possible, and to carve out time for yourself. You may know that you will always be available FOR your children when they need you, but what they remember is whether or not you were WITH them. Don't get too caught up in the "little stuff" like a child's messy hair, dirty play clothes, or an imperfect house. Worry about the things your child needs, such as a balanced diet, positive human interaction, daily physical activity, and time with you.

Demands of family, outside interests, and career call for multi-tasking; multi-tasking leads to stress! I would advise young women to focus on family activities and healthful lifestyles for the family. The other part of balance is giving yourself time for retreat. Finding the center so that you are spiritually and emotionally healthy allows you to be the best mother, wife, and professional you can be. An example of finding the balance that works for her family is my daughter, who is currently in a job that pays far less than she once made, but gives her weekends and late afternoons/evenings with her young children. She says it's a matter of priorities: she can work herself to a frenzy and make money now, but she would be sacrificing time with them. She can rear her children only once; she can make more money later. In a world that places so much emphasis on acquiring wealth and things, that is a hard decision to make. But there is no real balance without setting priorities.

Taking care of physical, mental, and emotional health is a life-long activity. As children leave the nest, women should be prepared to spend more time pursuing new interests, making friends, and reconnecting with friends and family members who are also transitioning to a quieter house, fewer mouths to feed, and retirement. They also should work with health care providers as changes in their bodies present physical and emotional challenges and possibly affect personal relationships.

When I retired, I had the opportunity to be in a situation where the participants (most younger than I) were asked to create goals for their personal, spiritual, and professional lives. That exercise reinforced for me that I still had an opportunity to consciously address the direction of my life in retirement. I determined that my over-riding objective was to make a difference. Since then, I've engaged in purposeful living, whether I'm playing or attending to church/civic/family obligations.

So my advice is to laugh, dance, love freely, travel, make plans, keep learning, take up new hobbies, spend time with family and friends. To quote C.S. Lewis, "You are never too old to set a new goal or dream a new dream."

I believe wellness is total; it is physical, mental, emotional, and spiritual. Its manifestations are peace, happiness, contentment.

Elmarie Carr Brooks

Mrs. Elmarie Carr Brooks is a proud mother of four grown daughters and has been married to her husband for 43 years. Her entire life has been spent in a "nurturing" career. Mrs. Brooks works for the Starkville Public School District in Emerson Family Programs, strengthening families and helping single moms learn parenting skills. Before that, she was a daycare director and worked extensively with the Girl Scouts United States of America. She is an inspiring African American woman who has arguably helped more families in our community than any single other woman with her mixture of high expectations and patient love. In her spare time, she loves to go fishing, travel, spend time with family, and teach the children's sermon at her church. She plans to retire in a few years so she can fit in more of the things she loves to spend time doing in her free time. Here is her wisdom:

* * *

Growing up, I always wanted twelve children. That shows you how I feel about nurturing people, and it drove my career toward helping professions. I was the first member of my family to graduate from college, and I wanted to use my education to help others.

I think the key to helping other people is to model the behavior we want others to have. If we want to create healthy, happy people, we have to show them how to live that way, not just tell them. I think that is one of the biggest mistakes we make as adults, parents, or leaders in the church. We tell young people what to do, but we do the opposite. We tell them to eat properly, but we eat junk.

We do not show them what health looks like. I notice that even at events that are supposed to be healthy, like church events, we are bringing more and more fast and unhealthy foods. We have to figure out how to change that culture without making enemies of each other. Being a model for your children, your neighbor's children, and your church's children is the most important thing we can do for young girls regarding health. I am not saying it's easy. It is hard even in my own family, but we have to hold ourselves to the standards we want for our children. I think if we get out in front of it, we can change health dramatically by modeling what it looks like.

Our job as a parent is to prepare our children to thrive in a culture that is not set up in their best interest. You start by doing those right things first. Preparation includes making three healthy meals a day available and taking care of their basic health needs. I focus on teaching moms to take care of themselves first, because if you don't take care of your own health and exercise needs, you cannot take good care of your children. You have to schedule time to take care of yourself. Make it a priority. Write it down on the calendar: doctor's appointment, exercise, grocery shopping, women's group at church. Schedule and prioritize.

I go to home visits all the time where Mama is in the bed at 9:45 with the baby. Good care is not easy. It is exhausting giving good care, but you have got to get up out of that bed, put your clothes on, and do the right thing for your child even when you don't feel like it.

I work with a lot of single moms who are still living at home with their parents. We disable our children by enabling them. It does not help our children to let them behave in ways that are destructive.

When we prop up bad behavior as parents, we hurt our children by furthering that behavior. It stops our young people from growing up and becoming contributing members of society when we continue to treat them like small children. My advice is, if you don't have a job, you don't have a flat screen TV or a fancy phone!

My mom worked really hard and didn't have a lot of time. She was trying to pay bills and prepare food. My dad was there, but women did most of the parenting. She was so busy working that she did not always have time to talk things through with us, but what she did say stuck with us even when she was not there. She prepared the gardens where we grew fresh food. She taught us to keep a clean mind and a clean heart. She took us to church. She encouraged and supported us in the best way she knew how. It is important to me that moms do the best they can with what they've got. All moms can encourage their children, no matter their circumstances. Even busy moms can model good behavior for their children.

Read to your child every night. Talk to you children. Get on their eye level. Listen to them. Actively communicate with children. Let them finish their sentences. Value what they share with you. Acknowledge that you hear what they are saying. Paraphrase what they said to you. Let them know that you are interested in their voice, and start that early. Then, when they get to be thirteen, fourteen, and fifteen years old, they are going to come and say, "Mom, this is what's going on. I really need to talk to you."

I think women need to celebrate when they send their children out into the world. Just have fun! When all of my children were finally grown and gone, you talk about some relief! I finally had so much time to do the things I love. I get out and work in the yard, and if I don't want to cook a full meal, I don't have to. Our job, first, is to take care of, nurture, and provide for our children, but if you do a pretty good job of that then you should not be out there running around after them as adults. When your cycles stop coming, Hallelujah! Enjoy yourself in these twilight years. These are fantastic years.

Mental health is so important. I really think it prevents a lot of these diseases we are coming down with. A good, positive mindset and saying good, positive things to yourself and others is the best way to promote wellness for ourselves and our families. Enjoy life.

Look at all the information you have, make decisions, and if you mess up? Try again. Tomorrow is a new day. Don't hold on to things you cannot change. Choose to be around positive people who value positive things. Having strong values, being part of a strong family unit for added support, and avoiding negativity all contribute to wellness and a happy life.

Nancy Woodruff

I hold a Women's Wellness retreat each year at The Homestead Education Center. At last year's retreat we honored Nancy as a Wise Elder. A child of Mississippi, Nancy's quest for bringing about health and wholeness to her home state is unparalleled. Her quiet questioning, persistent pushing, and modest example have moved our corner of the world forward in health and post-feminism. "Coming home" is how Nancy teaches people how to heal the world. She feels that saving the earth begins in our kitchens. This is a radical and powerful idea that could only be carried off well by someone who has taken the time to live as Nancy has. Here is her wisdom:

* * *

As a culture, we need to question two things: the busyness of our lives and the levels of toxicity (endocrine-disruption) in our physical environments.

Regarding busyness: young girls (and boys) need adults in their daily lives who are less stressed, more able to be attentive, and available to give and receive affection and love. Young humans who are loved unconditionally are more able to love themselves.

Young girls who love themselves as a whole people will more naturally regard their sexuality in a positive way. Positive love from parents to girls needs to come early, ahead of the media and peer influences over which parents have less and less control as their children grow older.

Censorship/parental controls on inappropriate media can help, but we can't expect real change until culture changes. As wellness and personal health take more center stage in our lives, families will begin to function better, and media will begin to reflect this. Until then, each family unit does what it can to protect and

nurture its girls (and boys) toward healthy love and respect for themselves.

Regarding toxicity: chemical exposures are seldom linked in mainstream media to damaged hormonal and sexual function, but environmental and health science has begun to explain "endocrine-disruption." As we become more toxin and chemical aware as a culture, our environments will become cleaner. As we choose products more carefully at the personal and home level, toxicity levels will change, and young girls will have less exposure overall.

The only birth control available when I was a teen growing up in the 1960's was the church. Moral structures included boys but placed much more responsibility on girls, something inherent in most cultures across time.

If I could go back to that time, I would tell myself to learn the basics of physiology and function – things that were not part of education back then. I would have a conversation with myself about wellness and its connection to happiness. We thought not at all about wellness back then.

I wish young mothers would *value* everything they are doing to care for themselves and others, whether those around them value it or not. Realize that we humans have lost caregiving skills and have to regain them, so be patient with yourselves and keep learning and watching. Search for caregivers around you who are "naturals" and watch them. See how they think and how their attention is on what is needed in themselves and for others.

There is an ability in the natural caregiver to see through the eyes of the person in his or her care, to feel the world as the individual does, and to apply sound knowledge and skills to meeting the person's needs.

Learn yourself—using whatever tools appeal to you—and then listen more to who you are than to the culture around you. We are often led into doing things because culture programs us to do so, e.g. "women can have it all" now that we are liberated, college educations are essential, parental leave will solve the problem of having time at home with newborns, etc.

If your life and health are both out of balance, center down on your health for a while and simply maintain the basics of life until you've worked on health. With time, changes in your health will bring about a balance in your life as well.

It never stops—this need to care for our health. Make it second nature; *assume* that caring for yourself is the way the world works even if it is a skill you've had to acquire while those around you do otherwise. Accept aging with grace, but don't give up or put aside caring for yourself.

How we die depends on how we live—even until the last day. Good health is not about living forever; it's about living with as much function and comfort and joy and generosity and purpose as we can manage. This is perhaps the greatest influence and gift you can give those around you and those you will leave behind.

Women's twilight years can be the best years. You can be yourself more now than ever. You can wear and say and do more things just because they make sense *to you*. If you've not taken care of yourself before this time in life, then begin. It's never too late; the wrinkles and baggy skin may improve, or they may not. You'll still feel better; you'll have more inclination to heal family wounds, to be generous, and to love the next generation despite their flaws and failures.

We have almost lost our elders to dementia and chronic disease, but we need their wisdom more than ever. If you are entering your elder years, know that you have things to share, that you can make a difference despite the fast-paced world around you. Small things matter; the kindness of strangers matters; you don't have to be responsible for the world anymore, so relax. Then look around for what you can give and stay engaged as long as you possibly can.

Women's wellness means finding ways to know the uniqueness of ourselves and others as well as how to use our talents and strengths for the common good—family, planet, community; whatever we are drawn to make better. Well women are centered and balanced, they know life's journey will have ups and downs, and they are ready to learn and grow and have patience with others.

Women's wellness also means women recognizing and taking personal responsibility for the most awesome gift there is: the ability to bring human life into the world and to nurture it. When Women's Wellness really comes into its own, it will mean thinking ahead and knowing ourselves before having children and knowing how to connect with a partner wisely. The wellness of women—or the lack thereof—drives much of what happens around the globe. It is the center from which daily life is made better or worse and from which home is recognized for its value or not. From the power and strength of well women, everything changes: families thrive, business turns green, and health spreads outward to others.

* * *

These three women have lived long and well. They have much to teach us about how to create a good life as strong, healthy females. It is their stories and stories of many more women like them that need to be passed down in order to preserve this wisdom. There are key elements to creating a good life. We don't have to reinvent the wheel, but in our disconnected culture it often feels like we do.

Sharing our stories, our successes, our challenges is critical to transmitting a culture of wellness.

Chapter 14

Sustainable Wellness:
Heal Yourself; Heal Our Culture

"God gave us the gift of life; it is up to us to give ourselves the gift of living well."
                                                    —Voltaire

Living and living well are two very different things. I used to believe that all my physical and mental ailments happened to me and that I needed to get each part that bothered me "treated." What I believe now is that my behaviors, diet, and lifestyle determine how my body will react to things that cause disease, illness, or inflammation. Living well is not just something we have to leave up to luck or good genes.

The latest research demonstrates clearly that we can change our genes. Living well is our responsibility to ourselves and our families, but it takes a huge shift in lifestyle and how we understand illness. It is a shift away from a culture that fights disease toward a culture that cultivates wellness and sustains it. It is up to the Wise Elders who have successfully crossed through this terrain to reach back and share their maps with the rest of us.

While I am far from being wise, there are some things I have learned on my journey that I would like to share. There were lots of times while I struggled with vulvovaginal and mental illnesses that I told myself, "You have so many things going for you, just deal with the inconveniences you do have." When that didn't work, I tried to deal with my ailments individually on a symptom/treatment basis, which is what our culture teaches us. It is why there are hundreds of types of over-the-counter medicines specific to your symptoms. If you have a cold, you may need a decongestant or an antihistamine, or you may need fever relief, or maybe your sinuses are dry. What happened to eating chicken soup and taking a few days to recover? When did we shift so soundly away from building up our immune systems, rest, and fluids?

Until recently, I treated my children's symptoms the same way. We had the Little Noses for coughs, for fevers, for itchy eyes, or whatever other symptom you can think of. We bought drops for gas, for teething, for constipation. I bet we spent thousands of dollars on over-the-counter and prescription medicines in the first five years of my kids' lives.

What I am learning, and what I want to share, is that the symptoms of illness are always signs of something larger that is off-kilter in the body. Treating symptoms lets us live, maybe even symptom-free, but it won't let us live well. Symptoms keep coming back. They may go away for a while. They may change form slightly, but they always return if we don't support the underlying issues that cause symptoms.

I am beginning to understand that my ailments didn't just happen to me. They were signs from my body that something was wrong. They refused to quit sounding their alarms until I paid attention. I am amazed at the potential for living well now that I have finally woken up to the fact that the whole body is connected, not only to all its other parts, but also to the environment in which it exists. I am now 40 years old, and I feel better than I have since I was ten. I always assumed I would just have to make the best of my myriad female and mental issues. I was wrong. Living well is possible for me, and I believe it is possible for most people.

Living Well

In my search for solutions to particular female health issues, I realized the only way wellness could happen was if I had a healthy body, overall. So how do you get a healthy body? The truth is, it is hard! I don't mean that in the sense of killing yourself at the gym. I no longer belong to a gym because I am out in the garden and hiking with my kids. I mean hard in the sense of making health a priority in a culture that extols quick, cheap, and instant. Understanding of root cause issues, food, environmental factors, and spiritual and emotional impacts are the keys to good health across all the hundreds of books and articles I found on my journey. I have addressed these in almost every chapter. Identifying them is one thing. Making them happen in real life is a lot tougher.

Baby Steps

Making one small change is important. Making one small change gives you the confidence you need to make others. You don't have to change your entire existence right away; you just have to make one change. Here are a few:

- Find out *why* you need to make changes. Watch a video on Pop Tech with Dr. Dean Ornish called *Healthy Connections*. It is a great, short recap that explains what making changes can do for your health quickly.

- Find out *what* changes you can make that will have the biggest impact. Search Dr. Terry Wahls on TEDx for her talk, "Minding Your Mitochondria."

- Pick *one thing* on the list of changes you want to make. Don't do all of them. Health is a process. It isn't something you accomplish, check off, and put in the attic.

- *Forgive* yourself. If you screw up, and you will, don't beat yourself up. Let it go, and start again the next day. My rule of thumb is: for every two good days, I can have one off day.

- Make it about *joy*. You will never stick to a program or a plan that feels painful. It has to feel exciting, fun, *joyful*. And you know what? Feeling like you have energy, getting your creativity back, and seeing health ailments fade is exciting!

Here are some specific baby steps you could make based on the videos above:

1. Triple your intake of veggies a day. Start with adding one smoothie filed with leafy greens to your daily diet. Just this one change made a huge difference in my level of energy. My go-to-recipe: Blueberry Kefir (from the store), frozen blueberries, a handful of kale or spinach, and a little water.

2. Start eating one probiotic food every day. Probiotic pills are not as easily assimilated by the body. Learn to make one easy fermented food and eat a little every day.

3. Take a high quality fish oil or krill supplement.

4. Learn to meditate. Stress is at the top of the list for every major disease: heart disease, cancer, depression, and autoimmune disorders. The science behind benefits of meditations is astounding. There are guided mediations all over the internet. When I started, I couldn't sit quietly for five minutes, now I am up to fifteen with a guided meditation podcast.

5. Walk. Park at the back of the parking lot where your car will be safer. Take the stairs at work. Do two laps around your office after lunch. Just start moving a little bit.

My advice is to make small changes until you are ready to take the plunge. Change out sugar for honey. Buy a water bottle and fill it up four times a day. Double your intake of leafy greens. See if you can find a healthy replacement for soda. Start eating fermented foods daily. Pick one thing. You can do that. In order to make health a central part of our lives, my family had to have a pretty good reason. We had a few: Max, Ben, and Cecelia. We made our first health changes for them even before we cared enough to do it for ourselves. Baby steps are a good place to start.

Crowding Out

I don't really want a spinach, blueberry, and kefir smoothie for breakfast. What I want is biscuits and gravy. But, if I can think about how I will feel at two this afternoon, I choose the smoothie. If I eat the biscuits and gravy, at two o'clock, I will feel like I have no other earthy choice but to drop my head to my desk and sleep. Two o'clock is right before my kids get home, and I want to feel like spending time with them. If I eat the biscuits, I will literally drag myself through the second half of my day. If I eat the smoothie, I don't need a nap. If I eat the smoothie, I am much more likely to enjoy the hours with my kids after school. We are more likely to go outside, ride bikes, or go for a walk. If I eat the biscuits, we will probably sit around and play on our computers. I have to think about it like that.

Crowding out is my second tip for regaining health. Crowding out does not require you to give up anything; you just add in a whole lot of good things. Here is how it works. If you fill up 3/4 of your plate with vegetables, there is only 1/4 left for other things. If you eat a humongous salad for lunch, you don't have as much room for food that makes you feel bad. If you add walking 20 minutes each evening, you have less time to drink beer. It can be simple. Don't give up anything; just add in one or two commitments you can stand. Here are some suggestions:

- Increase your intake of organic vegetables every day. Go to the local farmers market, join a CSA (community supported agriculture where you buy a share in a farm and receive a box of veggies every week), plant a winter garden.

- Walk 20 minutes three times a week. Free. Done.

- Add a healthy smoothie to your breakfast; don't replace it yet, just add it.

- Add in a multivitamin and fish oil. Get the mercury free fish oil. Read reviews on vitamin companies. Invest in a good one.

- Add one pot of grass-fed chicken bone broth to your diet each week—this is so incredibly easy, and the health benefits are astounding. Roast a grass-fed, organic chicken for dinner in the oven. Take all the bones and carcass leftovers and throw them in the crock pot. Cover with spring water and add a few tablespoons of vinegar. Turn the crock pot on for 48 hours and walk away. Strain bone broth into jars and store in the fridge. When I cook rice, I use bone

236

broth instead of water. When I need a quick dinner, I pull out the bone broth and throw in whatever leftover veggies we have for soup.

- Learn to make one fermented food and work a little into your diet every day. I recommend Sandor Katz's *Wild Fermentation*.

- Add in a guided meditation every morning. There are tons of guided meditations on Sound Cloud and YouTube that take fifteen minutes a day. The research coming out on the health impacts of meditation is compelling. *Yoga Journal* has a list of online "Less than Five Minute Meditations."

Add in some healthy food and behaviors, and you'll have less time and space for your old, unhealthy ones. These changes will make sure you start to feel good again. Crowd out bad behaviors with good ones. It is hard to drink too much if you know you are getting up early to go walking. It is easier to skip dessert if you eat a humongous salad. It is even easier if you keep good quality chocolate in the house for occasions when you have a craving. Don't give up anything, just overdo the good stuff.

Elimination

Once you feel encouraged by the changes you have made, you might be ready to take another important step in healing: Elimination. Now, I know that name sounds terrifying to those of us with addictive behaviors. It causes our stomachs to clench up and kicks in our "I'm outta here" response mechanisms. But just hear me out.

Some women I know hosted a program called *21 Days to Bliss*, which those of us who participated jokingly called *21 Days to Hell*. This, along with the *Clean Gut Diet*, helped me over the hump. 21 Days is manageable. I thought, *I can do that!* Did I cheat? Yes. Did I fail some? Yes. But I stuck with it enough to get some incredible results. I stuck with it enough that two years later, it is still my way of life.

Here is how it works. Most of us eat crap. Seriously, the majority of Westerners pour a steady stream of inflammatory and unhealthy foods into our bodies year after year and wonder why we have so much chronic disease. Taking Baby Steps and Crowding Out some of these harmful foods begins to introduce nutrients we have been low in perhaps our whole lives. And that is good, but if we really want to heal and see dramatic results, we have to take out the foods that harm us, eventually.

Some of the foods that harm us are obvious: high fructose corn syrup, preservatives, food dyes, etc. Others are less so, and depend upon the person. The only way you can know what foods you are sensitive to is to take out all the food triggers, let your intestines heal, and then add them back in slowly, one at a time, to see what happens.

The seven most common irritants for people are: gluten, dairy, tree nuts, sugar and sugar substitutes, shellfish, eggs, and soy. Others include caffeine and night shade vegetables. This is tough; I am not going to lie. I documented my elimination struggles for myself and my daughter, and it was hard and fraught with failures. But here is the thing, it worked. I am coming up on my second year without antidepressants since I was twenty-two. My daughter overcame a severe sensory disorder (which recently reappeared the week after Halloween—no wonder).

I have become fascinated by stories of healing from people who have successfully eliminated foods that were either killing them or making their daily lives miserable. If you are ready to try an elimination diet, I recommend following a protocol at first. Try *Clean Gut*, or join a support group like 21 Days to Bliss. Do a three week cleanse. If you don't make it the first time, do it again. Feeling the benefits of health for a short time is life changing. People ask all the time how I have the willpower to stick to this diet, but it isn't due to willpower at all. I eat what I want to eat, and what I want to eat is food that makes me feel good! When you start to feel good, really good, for the first time, change becomes easier and long-term change becomes possible.

Root Causes

Understanding root causes means realizing that your symptoms, or your children's symptoms, point to a deeper imbalance. For example, my kids kept getting ear infections. I kept treating them with the pink antibiotic until they became immune to it and had to move on to a more powerful antibiotic.

When I learned about the connection between c-sections and a lack of beneficial bacteria in the gut, I was horrified at what I had done to my kids. The antibiotics killed the bad bacteria, but also any of the remaining good stuff they had left, and I wasn't replacing it, making them more susceptible to future infections.

Lack of beneficial bacteria in the gut is linked to so many symptoms. In essence, I was setting my kids up to deal with some of the same symptoms I was so frustrated with myself: hormonal problems, PMS, skin problems, prostate trouble, candida, anemia, some allergies, vitamin B deficiency, vaginal and bladder infections, irritable bowel syndrome, and osteoporosis, all common health problems associated with inadequate beneficial bacteria, according to Dr. David Williams, who has written about bacterial imbalance on drdavidwilliams.com.

Once we all started on foods high in probiotics and used antibiotics much more judiciously, the ear infections went away. Also, because I learned about probiotics shortly after the birth of our third child, she was sick much less often than the boys had been. She was also out of daycare for the first year of her life, but I believe the combination of factors, rather than genetic luck, made a difference. Once I understood that the yeast infections and the vulvodynia had nothing to do with my vagina and everything to do with the balance in my gut and the rest of my body, I was cured. Treating the symptoms didn't work. Creating a healthy body did.

Food

Once you understand that symptoms point to but are not themselves root causes of health issues, the next arena to take on is food. It is so simple, really; we are what we eat (and what we breathe and surround ourselves with). If that is true, then what we put into our body three times a day, or more, becomes central to our health.

What most Americans put into their bodies everyday is processed food high in corn syrup and carbs. I live in the state with the highest obesity rates and the highest rates of diabetes. We are eating absolute junk. Although it is an agricultural state, Mississippi has a high percentage of what are called "food deserts," which are populated areas with little or no food retail provision. Food deserts are most prevalent in the poorest areas. Convenience markets do not exist in nice neighborhoods. In my town, they serve as grocery stores for people without cars. However, even as a person who can drive to the grocery store, finding fresh, wholesome food is challenging.

Our local grocery recently expanded its two mini-aisles of natural foods to six. I almost did cartwheels! They added an organic vegetable section, and sometimes you can find organic strawberries. It isn't convenient to find healthy food, nor is it economical all the time, but it is vitally important.

This is my recipe for finding real food. First, there is a Facebook page a friend of mine started called Real Food Starkville. On it, they keep an up to date list of all the people in our community who produce and sell whole foods. On it you can find eggs, honey, chicken, beef, vegetables, and any number of other products. If your town doesn't have one of these, start one!

Second, we have a thriving farmers market in town thanks to the efforts of local volunteers who wanted to access local, healthy food. It started as a few trucks backed up on a corner. It has grown into a Saturday morning event, and recently, Tuesday evenings have been added.

Every town needs a farmers market. Don't wait for change to

happen; make it happen.

Third, we belong to two CSAs—community supported agriculture groups. In this model, participants buy a share of the farmers' business. In our case, we buy a share of a grass-fed cow and pig. When the animal has been processed, we pick up our share. There are vegetable CSAs that deliver a box of fresh produce to their members each week. I have even heard of herbal CSAs. In order to find one near you, check out *Local Harvest*, a nonprofit, online database that connects consumers with local farmers by zip code.

Fourth, we grow our own. Seven years ago, I didn't know how to grow a cucumber. Now we have a four-season garden that supplements the food we get locally.

We read, took classes, asked old-timers, and experimented. Everyone needs to know how to grow something.

What to Eat

I subscribe to a modified Paleo diet, high in vegetables. This is because our youngest child had a health crisis that led us to cut out nearly anything we thought could cause it in order to make her well. It worked, and we all felt better, so it stuck.

We aren't strict out of the house, and it did take several months to adjust to what we cooked, what we snacked on, and what we purchased, but now it is a way of life.

When I get "off," I start to feel groggy around two in the afternoon again. I start to crave sweets and carbs, and I'm more irritable around my periods and more moody, overall. On the diet, I am a different person. I am the person I always envied – full of energy and enthusiasm for things.

We eat all kinds of healthy meat: beef, pork, chicken. I buy the normal kid-friendly meals, only healthy, like organic hot dogs, organic (gluten free) chicken nuggets, and organic, phosphate-free cold cuts. But I am learning to cook meat in easy ways.

One of our favorite meals is a whole roasted chicken baked over three small oven-proof bowls filled with water and covered in sea salt. The chicken is pasture raised by a friend of ours, but the cooking method is easy. I am not a great cook, but I have learned a dozen easy, healthy meals, and we stick to those.

We eat all kinds of nuts and seeds for snacks with dried fruits. We eat every kind of vegetable under the sun. If I don't know how to cook it, I mix it into a smoothie to get it in my kids. We eat fruit in season when it is cheap, and we freeze it for when it is not. I hide vegetables in things like pancakes and waffles. Pamela's gluten free mix and a waffle maker have saved us on many meals. We sweeten everything with honey.

I have found a few tolerable gluten-free pastas we like, but mostly we cook rice in a rice cooker (again, we are modified on the Paleo). Lara Bars are a staple among my family. The most important thing I have learned is to read labels at the store. You should see my ten-year-old! He is a pro at picking something up, turning it over, and saying, "Nope, lots of stuff you can't pronounce."

What we don't buy is high fructose corn syrup. There are very few things that come pre-packaged that do not contain corn syrup. Everything from salad dressing to catsup to baked beans has it. We don't eat food coloring, which is in almost every kid-marketed food. My daughter and I don't eat gluten. We eat some dairy. Hard cheeses that have been aged a long time are safe; pasteurized milk is not for us. We drink almond milk like crazy. No one complains anymore. I cook with cultured butter, ghee, or coconut oil.

This has all been quite a switch for us. It felt impossible at first. We messed up a lot. We still have a hard time sticking to it when we go out of town or even out to dinner. Thankfully, none of us has a food intolerance so severe that we have to be strict, and we can have a sense of humor about our lifestyle change. One of my favorite scenes from our shift in food was walking into the kitchen where my boys had found an old package of flour tortillas that had fallen down behind the drawers in the fridge. They were devouring them. Ben said proudly, "Mom, we found gluten!"

I don't know that Paleo is the answer for us, or that it is the answer for anyone else, but I do believe the answer lies in real foods, processed and prepared in healthy ways. My favorite diet mantra comes from Michael Pollan: "Eat real food, not too much, mostly vegetables." I can remember that. I can work toward that. I can correct my course when I move away from that, and most importantly, I see results when I follow that advice.

Environment

"We are what we eat and what we breathe and surround ourselves with," is what I said in the last section. We are only beginning to understand how our environmental surroundings impact our overall health. These are scary issues because they are so hidden. I used to think that if you didn't live next door to a factory puffing out smoke, your environment was clean.

The things we bring into our homes by way of our cleaners, our carpets, and our personal care products have big influences on the way our bodies work. We cannot possibly avoid all of them. The best strategy is to become aware of the choices we have, when we do have them, and to protect our bodies' defense systems.

I clean with vinegar. We dropped our fabric softener. We changed all our personal care products to natural ones. I took a class on making homemade, natural cleaners and homemade personal care products, and I look up recipes on the internet. There are huge savings if you make these things yourselves.

We also eat lots of superfoods to counteract the bad elements that sneak in anyway. We belong to the Environmental Working Group, a non-profit that does extensive research on the toxicity of products. I have to tell myself on this one, "Do your best, but you cannot totally avoid them. Human bodies are resilient and can withstand quite an impact before they fold."

Spiritual and Emotional Awareness

I went to a talk at a convention last year on mindfulness. The teacher asked, "When you decide to cure yourself of some ailment, you reach for the medicine. Do you even check in with your body first? Do you even ask, 'Body, what's going on with you?'" Checking in, noticing the body, then noticing the breath is so simple, yet we rarely do it. That is all meditation or mindfulness is: checking in with the body, noticing the breath. Meditation and stress reduction are now listed as protocol among even the most traditional health centers in the country.

When I was researching my own health, I was startled and frustrated by how many places like Johns Hopkins and the Mayo Clinic listed meditation as a possible treatment.

This is what Mayo states:

> **Meditation might also be useful if you have a medical condition, especially one that may be worsened by stress.**
>
> **While a growing body of scientific research supports the health benefits of meditation, some researchers believe it's not yet possible to draw conclusions about the possible benefits of meditation.**
>
> **With that in mind, some research suggests that meditation may help people manage symptoms of conditions such as anxiety disorders, asthma, cancer, depression, heart disease, high blood pressure, pain, and sleep problems.**

In the early stages of my quest for health I thought, "They just don't know what to do about vaginas, so they tell people to meditate because they know it can't hurt and they have to say something!"

I didn't put much stock in meditation, mindfulness, or prayer as it related to healing the body. I went to church every Sunday. I prayed regularly and said blessings before meals, but I gravely underestimated the power of faith and meditative practice as they relate to health and wellness.

I always understood the "placebo effect" to mean that people were given a fake versus a real drug. Placebo equaled fake, trick, not real. My husband explained it differently to me, based on his studies in medicine. Placebo is the mind's ability to heal the body. It is the body's ability to heal itself because it thinks it can. This ability is real and documented. It clicked for me when Mike said, "Never underestimate the power of placebo."

I have volunteered to lead a senior yoga class once a week for the last three years at my church. It is not a church-related activity, and so we do not talk about God or Jesus or any other religiosity, but it most certainly is spiritual.

Every week, women with various aches, pains, and ailments from replaced hips to bulging discs, begin moving, stretching, breathing, and strengthening. I have witnessed incredible healing in that class. All we do is take time to pay attention, notice, laugh, and breathe.

Cutting edge pain management clinics are recognizing the benefits of mindfulness, and harnessing it. Surely we can open up our minds about these practices if the leading medical clinics have, and begin implementing them into our daily lives. Wake up ten minutes early and read a devotional. Take fifteen minutes out of your lunch break to breathe. Walk outside whenever you can. Take the foolish leap in your mind that it takes to believe it just might make a difference. What do you have to lose?

Changing the World from the Inside Out

When I was younger, I spent a lot of time and energy trying to change the world. Today, I believe the way to change the world is to change ourselves. Our vaginas exist within the larger context of our bodies. Our bodies exist within the larger context of our cultures. Start with you and move out. Make small, manageable changes. Eat a vegetable with every meal. Be the mom who hosts the healthy birthday party. When the bottle of cleaner runs out, replace it with vinegar and baking soda. Go to synagogue, take a yoga class, or read a meditation book. Try an alternative approach to your next illness. Talk to your kids honestly about sex. Help your children cultivate a healthy sexuality. Reinstate rites of passage. Ask your doctor hard questions. Read anything you can get your hands on. And share your story.

Most of all, don't be afraid to look foolish for your health. We need people who are not scared of drawing attention to themselves as they reject the "junk" culture we have inherited.

The world's health depends on lots of individuals taking a stand within their own homes, families, and communities. We get to determine the culture our children will inherit. I hope you will join me in rejecting a culture that treats and fosters disease and help me start creating a culture that cultivates wellness. As the inspirational Dr. Terry Wahls concludes her Tedx talk, "We could all herald in an epidemic of health. Because every day, you, all of you, choose what you eat and what you do. Now that you know, what choices will you make?"

Resources

My Favorite Books on Healthy Eating

Wild Fermentation: The Flavor, Nutrition, and Craft of Live-Culture Foods (2003) by Sandor Ellix Katz and Sally Fallon – learn just a few of the easy recipes in this book to start healing your gut lining.

The Wahls Protocol: How I Beat Progressive MS Using Paleo Principles and Functional Medicine (2014) by Terry Wahls M.D. and Eve Adamson. If you are already suffering from an autoimmune disorder, this one is a game changer.

*Grain Brain: The Surprising Truth about Wheat, Carbs, and Sugar-- Your Brain's Silent Killers (*2013) by David Perlmutter and Kristin Loberg. Doubtful about the hype around gluten? This one is a must read. My health journey started here.

Clean Gut: The Breakthrough Plan for Eliminating the Root Cause of Disease and Revolutionizing Your Health (2013) by Alejandro Junger – a practical guide for those of you ready to take the plunge into healthy living. Start with the 21 day cleanse in this book.

Resources for Forming Healthy Girls

Reviving Ophelia: Saving the Selves of Adolescent Girls (2005) by Mary Pipher, Ph.D.- #1 *New York Times* Bestseller and the groundbreaking work that poses one of the most provocative questions of a generation: what is happening to the selves of adolescent girls?

Beautiful Girl App—Dive inside to Dr. Christiane Northrup's *Beautiful Girl* to learn this simple but important message: to be born a girl is a very special thing and carries with it magical gifts and powers that must be recognized and nurtured. Explore pictures, learn new vocabulary, and personalize the story with your own narration. Through these empowering words and illustrations, little girls will learn how their bodies are perfect just the way they are.

Curricula by Kesa Kivel including: Girl House and Beyond and Moon Magic Workshops on Puberty - The curricula on this website are intended for use by facilitators working to educate girls and young women on gender and other issues in order to 1) help them become more aware, confident, compassionate, and empowered, and 2) help them cherish and celebrate being female.

Our Whole Lives: Honest, accurate information about sexuality changes lives. It dismantles stereotypes and assumptions, builds self-acceptance and self-esteem, fosters healthy relationships, improves decision making, and has the potential to save lives. For these reasons and more, we are proud to offer Our Whole Lives, a comprehensive lifespan sexuality education curricula for use in both secular settings and faith communities.

Favorite Resources on Women's Health:

Down There: Sexual and Reproductive Health the Wise Woman Way (Wise Woman Herbal Series) (2011) by Susun S. Weed and Alan McKnight This is an herbal guide to women's health. I love having home-based solutions to try before I run to the doctor. I also love Susan Weed's beautiful take on womanhood.

Dr. Kelly Brogan's Website (kellybroganmd.com)- Holistic women's health psychiatry focused on the identification of root causes of symptoms and natural treatments for whole body wellness. Perinatal nutrition, lifestyle, and environmental medicine considerations for mom and baby.

Women's Bodies, Women's Wisdom (Revised Edition): Creating Physical and Emotional Health and Healing (2010) by Christiane Northrup M.D. Northrup is comprehensive in her coverage of women's health issues in this book. I believe she gives a fairly balanced view of options for care.

Laura Horowitz Lehrhaupt V e-booklet. Larua is an advocate for healing vulvodynia and has written an e-book based on her experience of healing. She will send it to you at no charge if you email her bewelllaural@gmail.com.

What Your Doctor May Not Tell You About Menopause: The Breakthrough Book on Natural Hormone Balance (2004) by John R. Lee (Author), Virginia Hopkins (Author). I love this whole series and find it practical and helpful on so many topics.

Integrative Women's Health (2010) by Victoria Maizes (Editor), Tieraona Low Dog (Editor). This is a great place to start for healing women's issues.

Heal Pelvis Pain: The Proven Stretching, Strengthing, and Nuitrition Program for Relieving Pain, Incontinence, & I.B.S., and Other Symptoms Without Surgery by Amy Stein. Useful for women who cannot afford to pay for physical therapy.

Resources for Menopause Years

The Wisdom of Menopause (Revised Edition): Creating Physical and Emotional Health During the Change (2012) by Christiane Northrup M.D.

What Your Doctor May Not Tell You About Premenopause: Balance Your Hormones and Your Life From Thirty to Fifty (1999) by John R. Lee and Jesse Hanley

The Toa of Turning 50: What Every Woman In her 40s Needs to Know (2012) by Jennifer Boire's- Every woman in her 40s needs to read this book. Practical and spiritual, this book reframes perimenopause.

Resources for Natural Mental and Emotional Health

The Last Best Cure: My Quest to Awaken the Healing Parts of My Brain and Get Back My Body, My Joy, and My Life (2013). Donna Jackson Nakazawa. One of my all-time favorites for practical ways to regain joy.

Childhood Disrupted: How Your Biography Becomes Your Biography and How You Can Heal (2015). Donna Jackson Nakazawa. If you are serious about healing emotional trauma to impact physical health, this book is full of hope and practical tools.

Radical Acceptance (2004). Tara Brach. Tara has a great website and guided meditations. Her books are incredibly helpful for learning to live well with chronic conditions.

Unstuck: Your Guide to the Seven-Stage Journey Out of Depression **(2009)** by James S. Gordon M.D. – a great step-by-step for moving out of depression.

The Chemistry of Calm: A Powerful, Drug-Free Plan to Quiet Your Fears and Overcome Your Anxiety (2010) by M.D. Henry Emmons M.D. – great for people who are ruled by anxiety more than depression.

The Mood Cure: The 4-Step Program to Take Charge of Your Emotions (2003) by Julia Ross (Author) – Looking into amino acid therapy for a natural solution to depression is worthwhile for women trying to get off antidepressants.

Companies I Trust

Herbs – Mountain Rose Herbs - Mountain Rose Herbs offers high quality organic bulk herbs, gourmet spices, loose leaf teas, essential oils, herbal extracts, and natural body care ingredients. Their extensive selection includes certified organic, fair trade, ethically wild harvested, & Kosher certified botanical products. www.mountainroseherbs.com

Nutritional Supplements – Metagenics – Metegenics is a nutrition company founded by Dr. Jeffery Bland, a nutritional biochemist. This company is certified by outside agencies and is rigorous in their research and quality. http://www.metagenics.com/

Food sensitivity testing – Enterolab – This lab offers testing for sensitivities to foods and genetic testing to determine if you are at high risk for developing food sensitivities. www.enterolab.com

Websites I Like

Holistic Women's Health Psychiatry by Kelly Brogan, M.D. www.kellybroganmd.com - for an alternative approach to women's health with a scientific background, this is a comprehensive site.

Green Med Info www.greenmedinfo.com. One of the most comprehensive alternative medicine sites available.

Environmental Working Group www.ewg.org. EWG's mission is to empower people to live healthier lives in a healthier environment. They provide the dirty dozen list of most toxic foods each year, the list of highest mercury containing fish, and information on all kinds of products and their toxic loads. I love this group for the important work they are doing.

Bibliography

Chapter 1

Hanley, R. (1997). New Jersey Charges Woman, 18 With Killing Baby Born at Prom. Retrieved from: http://www.nytimes.com/1997/06/25/nyregion/new-jersey-charges-woman-18-with-killing-baby-born-at-prom.html

Rape, Abuse & Incest National Network (RAINN). (2009). How often does sexual assault occur? Retrieved from: www.rainn.org/get-information/statistics/frequency-of-sexual-assault.

Centers for Disease Control and Prevention (CDC). (2011). 2010 Sexually Transmitted Diseases Surveillance. Retrieved from: www.cdc.gov/std/stats10/adol.htm.

Jung, Carl. *The Archetypes—The Collective Unconscious* (collected works of Carl Jung, 1981) and Collective.

Chapter 2

Mary Pipher, Ph.D. (2005). *Reviving Ophelia: Saving the Selves of Adolescent Girls*. New York: Penguin.

WebMD. (n.d.) Vulvodynia: Causes, Symptoms, and Treatments. Retrieved from: www.webmd.com/women/guide/vulvodynia.

Chapter 3

Northrup, C.. (2010). *Women's Bodies, Women's Wisdom (Revised Edition): Creating Physical and Emotional Health and Healing*. Bantam.

Grish, K. (2005). Dealing with PMS: The Benefits of Being Premenstural. *Women's Health*. Retrieved from: www.womenshealthmag.com/health/pms/benefits..

Mayo Clinic Staff. (2014). Premenstrual Syndrome (PMS). Retrieved from: www.mayoclinic.org.

New York Times Health Guide. (2013). Premenstrual Syndrome. Retrieved from: www.nytimes.com/health/guides/disease/premenstrual-syndrome/causes.html.

Mayo Clinic Staff. (2014). Premenstrual Syndrome (PMS): Treatments and Drugs. Retrieved from: www.mayoclinic.org.

Office on Women's Health. (2012). Menstruation and the menstrual cycle fact sheet. Retrieved from: www.womenshealth.gov/publications/our-publications/fact-sheet/menstruation.html.

Bradley, L. (n.d.). Menstrual Dysfunction. *Cleveland Clinic Center for Continuing Education.* Retrieved from: http://www.clevelandclinicmeded.com/medicalpubs/diseasemanagement/womens-health/menstrual-dysfunction/.

Oz, M. (2009). Balance Your Hormones. *Oprah Health and Wellness.* Retrieved from:

Brogan, K. (2013, November 23). Resolve PMS to Prevent Postpartum Depression. [Web log comment]. Retrieve from: http://kellybroganmd.com/article/resolve-pms-prevent-postpartum-depression/.

Baker, S. (2012). Peace out, PMS! Natural cures for moodiness, soreness, and out-of-control cravings that come before that time of the month. *Women's Health.* Retrieved from: http://www.womenshealthmag.com/health/natural-pms-cures.

Chapter 4

Weed, S. S. (2011). *Down There: Sexual and Reproductive Health the Wise Woman Way.* Woodstock, NY: Ash Tree Publishing.

Hyman, Mark, M.D. (2010). How to Eliminate PMS in 5 Simple Steps. Retrieved from: http://drhyman.com/blog/2010/09/17/how-to-eliminate-pms-in-5-simple-steps/.

Centers for Disease Control and Prevention (CDC). (2014). *Human Papillomavirus (HPV):Genital HPV Infection - Fact Sheet.* Retrieved from: http://www.cdc.gov/std/hpv/stdfacthpv.htm.

Centers for Disease Control and Prevention (CDC). (2014). Human Papillomavirus (HPV): Genital HPV Infection - Prevention. Retrieved from: http://www.cdc.gov/hpv/prevention.html.

Brogan, K. & Ji, S. (2014, March 23). HPV Vaccine Maker's Study Proves Natural HPV Infection .

Beneficial, Not Deadly. *Green Med Info*. Retrieved from: http://www.greenmedinfo.com/blog/hpv-vaccine-maker-s-study-shows-natural-hpv-infection-beneficial-not-deadly.

Mercola, J. M.(2013, July 16). Oncology Dietitian Exposes Fraud in CDC's HPV Vaccine Effectiveness Study. Retrieved from: http://articles.mercola.com/sites/articles/archive/2013/07/16/hpv-vaccine-effectiveness.aspx.

Marie, J. (2013, April 17). In Our Hook-Up Culture, Why Can't We Talk About STDs? *Takepart*.

Bancroft, Dr. John (Director of the Kinsey Institute at Indiana University). "The Medicalization of female sexual dysfunction: the need for caution." http:www.ncbi.nlm.nih.gov/pmc/articles/PMC1124933/

Chapter 5

Retrieved from: http://www.takepart.com/article/2013/04/17/why-STDs-are-still-a-shameful-secret.

Weil, A. (2014). Chlamydia. *Condition Care Guide*. Retrieved from: http://www.drweil.com/drw/u/ART02959/Chlamydia.html.

Mayo Clinic Staff. (2014). Sexually transmitted diseases (STDs): Prevention. Retrieved from:
http://www.mayoclinic.org/diseases-conditions/sexually-transmitted-diseases-stds/basics/prevention/con-20034128.

University of Maryland Medical Center. (2012). Sexually transmitted diseases. Retrieved from:
http://umm.edu/health/medical/altmed/condition/sexually-transmitted-diseases.

Weed, S. S. (2012, March 3). Herbal Remedies for Three 'Collegiate' STIs/STDs. *The Edge*. Retrieved from:
http://www.edgemagazine.net/2012/03/herbal-remedies-for-stds/.

University of Maryland Medical Center. (2012). Sexually transmitted diseases. Retrieved from:
http://umm.edu/health/medical/altmed/condition/sexually-transmitted-diseases.

WebMD. (2003). Long-Term Stress May Trigger Herpes Outbreaks. Retrieved from:
herpes-outbreaks.

Webmd.com/balance/stress/management/news/19991111/lonf-term-atress-trigger-hwepwa-outbreaks.

Retrieved from: http://www.mdjunction.com/forums/genital-herpes-discussions/general-support/10381838-how-i-cured-my-genital-herpes

Enough is Enough: Making the Internet Safer for Children and Families. (2013). *Pornography Statistics*. Retrieved from: http://www.internetsafety101.org/Pornographystatistics.htm.

Hunt, J. (2012, March 9). Why the Gay and Transgender Population Experiences Higher Rates of Substance Use. *Center for American Progress*. Retrieved from: https://www.americanprogress.org/issues/lgbt/report/2012/03/09/11228/why-the-gay-and-transgender-population-experiences-higher-rates-of-substance-use/.

Centers for Disease Control and Prevention. (2014). Lesbian, Gay, Bisexual, and Transgender Health: LGBT Youth. Retrieved from: http://www.cdc.gov/lgbthealth/youth.htm.

Positive Images. (2014). For Parents: Questions and Answers. Retrieved from: http://www.posimages.org/resources/for-parents-questions-and-answers/.

Shore, J. (2014, May 29). Southern Baptist pastor accepts his gay son, changes his church. [Web log entry]. Retrieved from: http://www.patheos.com/blogs/johnshore/2014/05/southern-baptist-pastor-accepts-his-gay-son-changes-his-church/#ixzz3LiQvvNlb http://www.patheos.com/blogs/johnshore/2014/05/southern-baptist-pastor-accepts-his-gay-son-changes-his-church/.

Bason R., et al. "Report of the International Consensus Development Conference on Female Sexual Dysfunction: Definitions and Classifications," *Journal of Urology* (March 2000), 163:888–895.

Berman, L. (2013). How Childhood Abuse Can Manifest in Adult Relationships. *Everyday Health*. Retrieved from: http://www.everydayhealth.com/sexual-health/dr-laura-berman-childhood-abuse-and-adult-relationships.aspx.

Chapter 6

Gagos, S. (2006). Introduction. In *My Voice of Truth*. Retrieved from: http://www.myvoiceoftruth.com/mystory.html.

Mayo Clinic Staff. (2012, November 1). Yeast infection (vaginal): Treatments and Drugs. Retrieved from: http://www.mayoclinic.org/diseases-conditions/yeast-infection/basics/treatment/con-20035129.

Mayo Clinic Staff. (2014, July 17). Vulvodynia: Treatments and Drugs. Retrieved from: http://www.mayoclinic.org/diseases-conditions/vulvodynia/basics/treatment/con-20020326

Thackray, L. (2014, October 9). Ten years of agony, two operations and the prospect of never having children: Young woman's fight to get new drug used to treat her excruciating condition in Australia. *Daily Mail Australia.* Retrieved from: http://www.dailymail.co.uk/news/article-2738238/For-nearly-10-years-told-pain-head-But-23-year-old-Syl-never-able-kids-s-desperate-bring-new-treatment-excruciating-condition-Australia.html#ixzz3LivVS87s.

Mayo Clinic Staff. (2014, January 2). Interstitial cystitis: Treatments and Drugs. Retrieve from:
http://www.mayoclinic.org/diseases-conditions/interstitial-cystitis/basics/treatment/con-20022439.

Leger, A. (2009, November 2). Is PCOS a Symptom of a Gluten-Sensitivity or Celiac Disease? *The Savvy Celiac.* Retrieved from: http://www.thesavvyceliac.com/2009/11/02/is-pcos-a-symptom-of-a-gluten-sensitivity-or-celiac-disease/.

Hudson, T. (2006, October 17). Uterine Fibroids – Women's Health Update. [Web log comment].

Retrieved from: http://drtorihudson.com/articles/uterine-fibroids-womens-health-update/

Mayo Clinic Staff. (2013, May 18). Chronic pelvic pain in women: Treatments and Drugs. Retrieved from:
http://www.mayoclinic.org/diseases-conditions/chronic-pelvic-pain/basics/treatment/con-20030924.

Batha, E. (2013, September 29). Special report: The punishment was death by stoning. The crime?

Having a mobile phone. *The Independent.* Retrieved from: http://www.independent.co.uk/news/world/politics/special-report-the-punishment-was-death-by-stoning-the-crime-having-a-mobile-phone-8846585.html.

Chapter 7

Rios, T. (2014). Teen Pregnancy Rates Around the World. *Knoji*. Retrieved from: https://teens-teenagers.knoji.com/teen-pregnancy-rates-around-the-world/.

BBC Ethics Guide. (2014). Moral case against contraception. Retrieved from:

http://www.bbc.co.uk/ethics/contraception/against_1.shtml

BBC Ethics Guide. (2014). Contraception. Retrieved from

http://www.bbc.co.uk/ethics/contraception/

Planned Partenthood. Outercourse. Retrieved from:

http://www.plannedparenthood.org/health-info/birth-control/outercourse.

Mike. (2012, November 30). 4 Cool Statistics About Abstinence in the USA. *Waiting Till Marriage*. Retrieved from:

http://waitingtillmarriage.org/4-cool-statistics-about-abstinence-in-the-usa/.

Hutchcraft, R. (2012). 10 Ways to Practice Purity. *Christianity Today*. Retrieved from: christianitytoday.com/iyf/hottopics/sexabstinence/10-ways-to-practice-purity.html

Reem, U. (2011, June 15). Parenting Series Part VIII: Sexual Activities Beyond the "Norm" – What Should We Teach Our Teens. *Muslim Matters*. Retrieved from:

http://muslimmatters.org/2011/06/15/sexual-activities-beyond-the-norm-what-should-we-teach-our-teens/.

Brogan, K. (2013, February 8). That Naughty Little Pill: Birth Control Side Effects. [Web log entry.] Retrieved from:

http://kellybroganmd.com/article/that-naughty-little-pill-birth-control/.

Chapter 8

Evolving Wellness: Holistic, Natural, and Green Approach to Optimal Wellness. (n.d.) Review: Pearly & Lady Comp Natural Birth Control Contraceptive Devices. Retrieved from:

http://www.evolvingwellness.com/essay/review-pearly-lady-comp-natural-birth-control-contraceptive-devices.

Gurevich, R. (2014). 7 Things Every Woman Needs to Know About Fertility. Retrieved from:

http://infertility.about.com/od/tryingtoconceive101/a/Things-Every-Woman-Needs-To-Know-About-Her-Fertility.htm.

Chandra, A., Copen, C. E., & Stephen, E. H. (2013). Infertility and Impaired Fecundity in the United States, 1982–2010: Data From the National Survey of Family Growth. *National Health Statistics Reports, 67*. Retrieved from: http://www.cdc.gov/nchs/data/nhsr/nhsr067.pdf.

Infertility and In Vitro Fertilization. (n.d.). In *WebMD Reference*. Retrieved from:
http://www.webmd.com/infertility-and-reproduction/guide/in-vitro-fertilization.

British Broadcasting Corporation. (2014, September 24). IVF: the hope and despair - Claire's story. Retrieved from:
http://www.bbc.co.uk/devon/community_life/features/ivf_claires_story.shtml.

Wanjek, C. (2013, July 9). Can Acupuncture Help Women Get Pregnant? *Live Science*. Retrieved from:
http://www.livescience.com/38049-acupuncture-ivf-pregnancy-success.html.

Bouchez, C. (n.d.). The Ancient Art of Infertility Treatment. *WebMD*. Retrieved from:
http://www.webmd.com/infertility-and-reproduction/features/ancient-art-of-infertility-treatment.

Carpenter, L. (2009, October 24). The baby maker. *The Guardian*. Retrieved from:
http://www.theguardian.com/lifeandstyle/2009/oct/25/infertility-treatment-babies-doctor-zhai.

O-Pries, L. (2014, April 23). On infertility, grief, and hope. Spectrum. Retrieved from:
http://spectrum.yourbackline.org/fertility/on-infertility-grief-and-hope/.

Welcome. (n.d.). *Gateway Women*. Retrieved from: http://gateway-women.com/.

The Impact of The Environment on Your Fertility. (n.d.) *Fertility Factor*. Retrieved from:
http://www.fertilityfactor.com/helping_conception_environment.html.

Marchegiani, J. (2014). Natural Remedies for Hormonal Imbalance, Infertility, PCOS and PMS.

Primal Docs. Retrieved from: http://primaldocs.com/opinion/natural-remedies-for-hormonal-imbalance-infertility-pcos-and-pms/.

Resolve: The National Infertility Association. (2014). Retrieved from: http://www.resolve.org/.

Smith, M.K. (2004). Nel Noddings, the ethics of care and education. In *The Encyclopaedia of Informal Education*. Retrieved from: http://infed.org/mobi/nel-noddings-the-ethics-of-care-and-education/.

Chapter 9

Mayo Clinic. (n.d.). Pregnancy week by week. Retrieved from: http://www.mayoclinic.org/healthy-living/pregnancy-week-by-week/in-depth/pregnancy-nutrition/art-20043844?pg=2.

Mercola, J.M. No-Nonsense Guide to a Naturally Healthy Pregnancy and Baby. Retrieved from:

http://articles.mercola.com/sites/articles/archive/2009/11/07/no-nonsense-guide-to-a-naturally-healthy-pregnancy-and-baby.aspx.

Brogan, K. (2014, April 14). Vitamin D for pregnancy depression. [Web log entry]. Retrieved from:

http://kellybroganmd.com/snippet/vitamin-d-pregnancy-depression/.

Boyles, S. (2010, May 4). High Doses of Vitamin D May Cut Pregnancy Risks. *WebMD Health News*. Retieved from: http://www.webmd.com/baby/news/20100504/high-doses-of-vitamin-d-may-cut-pregnancy-risk.

Melnick, M. (2012, May 17). 6 Healing Benefits Of Probiotics. Retrieved from:

http://foodmatters.tv/articles-1/6-healing-benefits-of-probiotics.

Hunt, P. (2011, September 20). Toxins All Around Us. *Scientific American*. Retrieved from:

http://www.scientificamerican.com/article/toxins-all-around-us/.

Office on Women's Health. (September 27, 2010). Pregnancy: Staying Healthy and Safe. Retrieved

from: http://womenshealth.gov/pregnancy/you-are-pregnant/staying-healthy-safe.html.

Kristof, N. (2012, May 2). How Chemicals Affect Us. *New York Times*. Retrieved from:

http://www.nytimes.com/2012/05/03/opinion/kristof-how-chemicals-change-us.html?_r=0.

Kirkpatrick, K. (2009, April 9). Antioxidants: Arm Yourself With Food. [Web log entry].Retrieved from: http://www.doctoroz.com/blog/kristin-kirkpatrick-ms-rd-ld/antioxidants-arm-yourself-food.

Zerbe, L. & Main, E. (n.d.). The Best & Worst Ways to Cook Your Vegetables. *Rodale News.* Retrieved from: http://www.rodalenews.com/how-cook-vegetables.

Mercola, J.M. (2009, January 6). 8 Natural Remedies That May Help You Sleep. Retrieved from: http://articles.mercola.com/sites/articles/archive/2009/01/06/8-natural-remedies-that-may-help-you-sleep.aspx.

Weed, S. (n.d.). Herbal Allies for Pregnancy Problems. Retrieved from: http://www.susunweed.com/Article_Pregnancy_Problems.htm.

Centers for Disease Control and Prevention. (2012). Home Births in the United States, 1990–2009. [Data file]. Retrieved from: http://www.cdc.gov/nchs/data/databriefs/db84.htm.

Childbirth Connection. (2013). Why Is the National U.S. Cesarean Section Rate So High? Retrieved from: http://www.childbirthconnection.org/article.asp?ck=10456.

Kresser, C. (n.d.). Natural childbirth VI: Pitocin side effects and risks. Retrieved from: http://chriskresser.com/natural-childbirth-vi-pitocin-side-effects-and-risks.

Kresser, C. (n.d.). Natural childbirth VII: C-section risks and complications. Retrieved from: http://chriskresser.com/natural-childbirth-vii-c-section-risks-and-complications.

Kamel, J. (n.d.) 13 Myths About VBAC. Retrieved from: http://vbacfacts.com/13-myths-about-vbac/.

Sarah Ockwell-Smith, The Fourth Trimester- AKA Why Your Newborn Baby is Only Happy in Your Arms. Retrieved from: http://sarahockwell-smith.com/2012/11/04/the-fourth-trimester-aka-why-your-newborn-baby-is-only-happy-in-your-arms/

Mayo Clinic. Retrieved from http://www.mayoclinic.org/diseases-conditions/postpartum-depression/basics/symptoms/con-20029130

Chapter 10

Afterschool Alliance. (2007). Afterschool Programs: Keeping Kids —
and Communities —Safe. *Afterschool Alert Issue Brief, 27.* Retrieved from:
http://www.afterschoolalliance.org/issue_briefs/issue_crimeib_27.pdf.

Cohn, D., Livingston, G. & Wang, W. (2014, April 8). After Decades
of Decline, A Rise in Stay-at-

Home Mothers. *Pew Research Social & Demographic Trends.*
Retrieved from: http://www.pewsocialtrends.org/2014/04/08/after-decades-
of-decline-a-rise-in-stay-at-home-mothers/.

Archetypes. (n.d.). In *Goddess Guide.* Retrieved from:
http://www.goddess-guide.com/archetypes.html.

Chapter 11

Zamora, D. (2005). Women's Top 5 Heath Concerns. *WebMD
Feature.* Retrieved from:
http://www.webmd.com/women/features/5-top-female-health-concern.

Stoppler, M.C. (2014). Diseases More Common in Women. *Medicine
Net.* Retrieved
from:http://www.medicinenet.com/womens_health/page4.htm.

Brown, H. (2009, October 26). Women's health problems doctors still
miss. *CNN Health.* Retrieved from:
http://www.cnn.com/2009/HEALTH/10/19/undiagnosed.women.problem/.

Harvard Medical School. (n.d.) Gender matters: Heart disease risk in
women. *Harvard Health*

Publications. Retrieved from:
http://www.health.harvard.edu/newsweek/Gender_matters_Heart_disease_ri
sk_in_women.htm

Ziegelstein, R.D. Depression and heart disease. (n.d.) Johns Hopkins
Medicine, Women's

Cardiovascular Health Center. Retrieved from:
http://www.hopkinsmedicine.org/heart_vascular_institute/clinical_services/
centers_excellence/womens_cardiovascular_health_center/patient_informati
on/health_topics/depression_heart_disease.html

Skarnulis, L. (2004). Silent Risk: Women and Heart Disease. *WebMD Feature.* Retrieved from:
http://www.webmd.com/heart-disease/features/women-more-afraid-of-breast-cancer-than-heart-disease.

American Cancer Society. (2014). *What are the key statistics about cervical cancer?* [Data file].

Retrieved from:
http://www.cancer.org/cancer/cervicalcancer/detailedguide/cervical-cancer-key-

Statistics. Luciani, S., Cabanes, A., Prieto-Lara, E. & Gawryszewski, V. (2013). Cervical and female breast cancers in the Americas: current situation and opportunities for action. *Bulletin of the World Health Organization.* (91)640-649. doi: http://dx.doi.org/10.2471/BLT.12.116699.

Sack, K. (2009, November 20). Screening Debate Reveals Culture Clash in Medicine. *New York Times.* Retrieved from:
http://www.nytimes.com/2009/11/20/health/20assess.html?_r=0.

Orenstein, P. (2013, April 25). Our Feel-Good War on Breast Cancer. *New York Times.* Retrieved
from: http://www.nytimes.com/2013/04/28/magazine/our-feel-good-war-on-breast-cancer.html?pagewanted=all.

Simon, S. (2014). *Cancer Statistics Report: Deaths Down 20% in 2 Decades.* [Data file]. Retrieved from:
http://www.cancer.org/cancer/news/cancer-statistics-report-deaths-down-20-percent-in-2-decades.

Cancer.org. (2014). Cancer Facts & Figures Cancer Facts & Figures 2014. [Data file]. Retrieved from:
http://www.cancer.org/research/cancerfactsstatistics/cancerfactsfigures2014/.

Agnew, V. (2014, April 21). Yale Cancer Center Studies Find Lifestyle Changes Improve Biomarkers Associated with Breast Cancer Recurrence and Mortality. *Yale Cancer Center.* Retrieved from:
http://medicine.yale.edu/cancer/news/article.aspx?id=7483.

Turner, K.A. (2014). *Radical remission: surviving cancer against all odds.* Harper One.

Iliades, Chris. (2013, January 23). *Stats and Facts About Depression in America*. [Data file.]

Retrieved from: http://www.everydayhealth.com/health-report/major-depression/depression-statistics.aspx.

Chapman, D.P., Perry, G.S., & Strine, T.W. (2005).The vital link between chronic disease and depressive disorders. *Prevention of Chronic Diseases* [serial online] Retrieved from: http://www.cdc.gov/pcd/issues/2005/

Pratt, L.A., Brody, D.J., & Gu, Q. (2011). Antidepressant use in persons aged 12 and over: United States, 2005–2008. *NCHS* [Data file]. Retrieved from: http://www.cdc.gov/nchs/data/databriefs/db76.htm.

Brogan, Kelly. (2013, November 22). The Taper. *Mad in America: Science, Psychiatry, and Community*. Retrieved from: http://www.madinamerica.com/2013/11/taper/.

WebMD. Diabetes Health Center. Type 1 Diabetes. Retrieved from: http://www.webmd.com/diabetes/guide/type-1-diabetes.

Nakazawak, D. J. (2009). The Autoimmune Epidemic

National Institutes of Health. Autoimmune disorders. (n.d.). In *Medline Plus*. Retrieved from:

http://www.nlm.nih.gov/medlineplus/ency/article/000816.htm.

Pollan, Michael (2013, May 13). Some of my best friends are germs. *The New York Times*. Retrieved from: http://www.nytimes.com/2013/05/19/magazine/say-hello-to-the-100-trillion-bacteria-that-make-up-your-microbiome.html?pagewanted=all.

University of Bristol. (2014, September 3). Scientists discover how to 'switch off' autoimmune diseases. *ScienceDaily*. Retrieved from: www.sciencedaily.com/releases/2014/09/140903092157.htm.

O'Rourke, M. (2013, August 26). What's wrong with me? *The New Yorker*. Retrieved from:

http://www.newyorker.com/magazine/2013/08/26/whats-wrong-with-me.

Chapter 12

Mayo Clinic Staff. (2013). Perimenopause. Retrieved from: http://www.mayoclinic.org/diseases-conditions/perimenopause/basics/definition/con-20029473.

National Osteoporosis Foundation. (n.d.). What Women Need to Know. Retrieved from: http://nof.org/articles/235

Office on Women's Health. (2010). Menopause. Retrieved from: http://www.womenshealth.gov/menopause/symptom-relief-treatment/menopausal-hormone-therapy.html.

National Cancer Institute. (2011). Menopausal Hormone Therapy and Cancer. Retrieved from: http://www.cancer.gov/cancertopics/factsheet/Risk/menopausal-hormones.

Norsigian, J (2011) Our Bodies, Ourselves.

National Osteoporosis Foundation (n.d.). Learn about Osteoporosis: Prevention and Healthy Living. Retrieved from: http://nof.org/learn/prevention.

Shah, A. (2013, September 27). 15 Tips To Balance Your Hormones (Hint: You Don't Need To Take Hormones!). *Mind Body Green.* Retrieved from: http://www.mindbodygreen.com/0-11099/15-tips- to-balance-your-hormones-hint-you-dont-need-to-take-hormones.html.

Griffin, J. Menopause from the Chinese Perspective. (n.d.). *The Spirit of Maat, 2 (11)*. Retrieved from: http://www.spiritofmaat.com/archive/-jun2/chinese.htm.

Weed, S. S. Menopausal Years, the Wise Woman Way. (n.d.). Retrieved from://www.susunweed.com/Article_Menopausal_Years.htm.

Shepperd, L. (2014, March 12). Menopausal Journey: A Rite of Passage. [Web log entry]. Retrieved from: http://www.menopausegoddessblog.om/2014/03/12/menopausal-journey-a-rite-of-passage/.

Chapter 13

Williams, D. (2014, February 26). Symptoms of Bacterial Imbalance in the Digestive System. Retrieved from: http://www.drdavidwilliams.com/symptoms-of-bacterial-imbalance/#axzz30bsSe0nv.

Mayo Clinic Staff (2014). Meditation: A Simple, Fast Way to Reduce Stress. Retrieved from: http://www.mayoclinic.org/tests-procedures/meditation/in-depth/meditation/art-20045858

About the Author

Dr. Alison Buehler began her career as a special education teacher and earned a doctorate in educational administration. Since switching gears to raise three children, she began a nonprofit organization with her husband, *The Homestead Education Center* that provides writing, retreats, and workshops on personal growth, health and wellness. She is married to radiologist Mike Buehler and lives with her family in Starkville, Mississippi on a small farm where they raise children, chickens, goats, vegetables, and bees. Her writing focuses on stories that hold the power to heal.

Made in the USA
Middletown, DE
24 November 2019